Psychiatric and Behavioral Emergencies

Editors

DICK C. KUO
VERONICA TUCCI

EMERGENCY MEDICINE CLINICS OF NORTH AMERICA

www.emed.theclinics.com

Consulting Editor
AMAL MATTU

November 2015 • Volume 33 • Number 4

ELSEVIER

1600 John F. Kennedy Boulevard ● Suite 1800 ● Philadelphia, Pennsylvania, 19103-2899

http://www.theclinics.com

EMERGENCY MEDICINE CLINICS OF NORTH AMERICA Volume 33, Number 4
November 2015 ISSN 0733-8627, ISBN-13: 978-0-323-41684-9

Editor: Patrick Manley
Developmental Editor: Casey Jackson

Emergency Medicine Clinics of North America (ISSN 0733-8627) is published quarterly by Elsevier Inc., 360 Park Avenue South, New York, NY, 10010-1710. Months of issue are February, May, August, and November. Business and Editorial Offices: 1600 John F. Kennedy Boulevard, Suite 1800, Philadelphia, PA 19103-2899. Customer Service Office: 6277 Sea Harbor Drive, Orlando, FL 32887-4800. Periodicals postage paid at New York, NY, and additional mailing offices. Subscription prices are $155.00 per year (US students), $315.00 per year (US individuals), $523.00 per year (US institutions), $220.00 per year (international students), $450.00 per year (international individuals), $642.00 per year (international institutions), $220.00 per year (Canadian students), $385.00 per year (Canadian individuals), and $642.00 per year (Canadian institutions). International air speed delivery is included in all *Clinics'* subscription prices. All prices are subject to change without notice. **POSTMASTER:** Send address changes to *Emergency Medicine Clinics of North America*, Elsevier Periodicals Customer Service, 11830 Westline Industrial Drive, St. Louis, MO 63146. Customer Service (orders, claims, online, change of address): Elsevier Periodicals **Customer Service, 11830 Westline Industrial Drive, St. Louis, MO 63146. Tel: 1-800-654-2452 (U.S. and Canada); 314-453-7041 (outside U.S. and Canada). Fax: 314-453-5170. E-mail: journalscustomerservice-usa@elsevier.com (for print support); journalsonlinesupport-usa@elsevier.com (for online support).**

Reprints. For copies of 100 or more of articles in this publication, please contact the Commercial Reprints Department, Elsevier Inc., 360 Park Avenue South, New York, NY 10010-1710. Tel.: 212-633-3874; Fax: 212-633-3820; E-mail: reprints@elsevier.com.

Emergency Medicine Clinics of North America is covered in *MEDLINE/PubMed (Index Medicus), Current Contents/Clinical Medicine, EMBASE/Excerpta Medica, BIOSIS, SciSearch, CINAHL, ISI/BIOMED*, and *Research Alert*.

Contributors

CONSULTING EDITOR

AMAL MATTU, MD, FAAEM, FACEP
Professor and Vice Chair, Department of Emergency Medicine, University of Maryland
School of Medicine, Baltimore, Maryland

EDITORS

DICK C. KUO, MD
Associate Professor, Section of Emergency Medicine, Department of Medicine, Baylor
College of Medicine, Houston, Texas

VERONICA TUCCI, MD, JD
Assistant Professor, Section of Emergency Medicine, Department of Medicine, Baylor
College of Medicine, Houston, Texas

AUTHORS

MICHAEL K. ABRAHAM, MD, MS
Clinical Assistant Professor, Department of Emergency Medicine, University of Maryland
School of Medicine, Baltimore, Maryland

NATHAN GOLD ALLEN, MD
Section of Emergency Medicine, Department of Medicine, Center for Medical Ethics and
Health Policy, Baylor College of Medicine, Houston, Texas

MOHAMMAD SHAMI ALZAHRI, MD, MSc
Section of Emergency Medicine, Center for Medical Ethics and Health Policy, Baylor
College of Medicine, Houston, Texas; King Saud University, Riyadh, Saudi Arabia

SHARADAMANI ANANDAN, MD
Assistant Professor, Department of Psychiatry, Baylor College of Medicine, Houston,
Texas

SARA ANDRABI, MD
Department of Medicine, Section of Emergency Medicine, Baylor College of Medicine,
Houston, Texas

PATRICK R. AQUINO, MD
Assistant Professor, Department of Psychiatry and Behavioral Medicine, Lahey Hospital
and Medical Center, Tufts University School of Medicine, Burlington, Massachusetts

BIANCA ASAN, MD
Section of Emergency Medicine, Ben Taub Hospital, Baylor College of Medicine, Houston,
Texas

ERIN AUFDERHEIDE, MD
Section of Emergency Medicine, Baylor College of Medicine, Houston, Texas

RAKEL C. BEALL, MD
Assistant Professor, Psychiatry and Behavioral Sciences, Baylor College of Medicine, Houston, Texas

CEDRIC DARK, MD, MPH
Assistant Professor Medicine, Emergency Medicine, Baylor College of Medicine, Houston, Texas

ELIZABETH H. DAVID, MD
Assistant Professor, Menninger Department of Psychiatry and Behavioral Sciences, Baylor College of Medicine, Houston, Texas

NATHAN DEAL, MD
Section of Emergency Medicine, Emergency Center, Ben Taub General Hospital, Baylor College of Medicine, Houston, Texas

ARACELI FLORES, PhD
Assistant Professor, Menninger Department of Psychiatry and Behavioral Sciences, Baylor College of Medicine, Houston, Texas

SPENCER GREENE, MD, MS, FACEP
Assistant professor, Departments of Medicine and Pediatrics, Sections of Emergency Medicine, Baylor College of Medicine, Houston, Texas

THIAGO C. HALMER, MD, MBA
Emergency Medicine Resident Physician, Baylor College of Medicine, Houston, Texas

JIN Y. HAN, MD
Assistant Professor, Menninger Department of Psychiatry and Behavioral Sciences, Baylor College of Medicine, Houston, Texas

MICHELLE HONG, MD, PharmD
Section of Emergency Medicine, Emergency Center, Ben Taub General Hospital, Baylor College of Medicine, Houston, Texas

S. KALRA, MD, MPH
Post-doctoral Fellow, Department of Research and Innovation, St Luke's University Health Network, Bethlehem, Pennsylvania

JEFFREY STEVEN KHAN, MD
Menninger Department of Psychiatry and Behavioral Sciences, Baylor College of Medicine, Houston, Texas

DICK C. KUO, MD
Associate Professor, Section of Emergency Medicine, Department of Medicine, Baylor College of Medicine, Houston, Texas

BENJAMIN LI, MD
Medical Director, Harris Health Substance Abuse Treatment Program; Assistant Professor, Menninger Department of Psychiatry, Baylor College of Medicine, Houston, Texas

ANU MATORIN, MD
Associate Professor, Menninger Department of Psychiatry and Behavioral Sciences, Neuropsychiatric Center, Ben Taub General Hospital, Baylor College of Medicine, Houston, Texas

NIDAL MOUKADDAM, MD, PhD
Medical Director, Stabilization, Treatment and Rehabilitation (STAR) Program for Psychosis; Assistant Professor, Menninger Department of Psychiatry and Behavioral Sciences, Baylor College of Medicine, Houston, Texas

KIMBERLY NORDSTROM, MD, JD
Department of Psychiatry, Denver Health Medical Center, University of Colorado School of Medicine, Denver, Colorado

EBELECHUKWU A. ODIARI, MD
Section of Emergency Medicine, Baylor College of Medicine, Houston, Texas

NATALIE PON, MD
Department of Psychiatry, Baylor College of Medicine, Houston, Texas

GALWANKAR SAGAR, DNB, MPH, FACEE, Diplomat. ABEM
Assistant Professor of Emergency Medicine, University of Florida, Jacksonville, Florida

NAVDEEP SEKHON, MD
Assistant Professor, Section of Emergency Medicine, Baylor College of Medicine, Houston, Texas

ASIM A. SHAH, MD
Associate Professor, Departments of Psychiatry and Behavioral Sciences, Community and Family Medicine, Neuropsychiatric Center, Ben Taub General Hospital, Baylor College of Medicine, Houston, Texas

KAYLIN SIEVER, MD
Section of Emergency Medicine, Baylor College of Medicine, Houston, Texas

VERONICA SIKKA, MD, PhD, MHA, MPH, FAAEM
Chief, Emergency Medicine, Orlando VA Medical; Associate Professor, Emergency Medicine, UCF School of Medicine, Orlando, Florida

ANDREA GAIL STOLAR, MD
Associate Professor, Menninger Department of Psychiatry and Behavioral Sciences, Baylor College of Medicine, Houston, Texas

ALEXANDER TOLEDO, DO, PharmD
Clinical Assistant Professor, Department of Child Health, Arizona Children's Center, University of Arizona College of Medicine, Phoenix, Arizona

MINA TRAN, MD
Section of Emergency Medicine, Department of Medicine, Baylor College of Medicine, Houston, Texas

VERONICA TUCCI, MD, JD
Assistant Professor, Section of Emergency Medicine, Department of Medicine, Baylor College of Medicine, Houston, Texas

GARY M. VILKE, MD
Department of Emergency Medicine Behavioral Emergencies Research (DEMBER) Lab;
Department of Emergency Medicine, UCSD Health System, San Diego, California

MICHAEL P. WILSON, MD, PhD
Department of Emergency Medicine Behavioral Emergencies Research (DEMBER) Lab;
Department of Emergency Medicine, UCSD Health System, San Diego, California

Contents

Patients presenting with behavior or psychiatric complaints may have an underlying medical disorder causing or worsening their symptoms. Misdiagnosing a medical illness as psychiatric can lead to increased morbidity and mortality. A thorough history and physical examination, including mental status, are important to identify these causes and guide further testing. Laboratory and ancillary testing should be guided by what is indicated based on clinical assessment. Certain patient populations and signs and symptoms have a higher association with organic causes of behavioral complaints. Many medical problems can present with or exacerbate psychiatric symptoms, and a thorough medical assessment is imperative.

Acutely agitated or psychotic patients are particularly challenging to manage in the emergency department. Often these patients present with little or no history, and an adequate assessment may initially be difficult because of the condition of the patient. This article discusses basic concepts regarding agitation, and the related management goals and strategies.

Present in all patient populations, altered mental status (AMS) is a common, but nonspecific emergency department (ED) presentation that can signify serious underlying pathology. Delirium is a more defined mental status change caused by another medical condition that carries a high morbidity and mortality if missed. However, ED physicians miss the condition in more than 50% of cases. The ED physician should maintain a high index of suspicion for delirium, because if missed in the ED, delirium is more likely to be missed on the floors as well. Management of delirium is directed toward treating the underlying course.

Depression is the most common psychiatric illness in the general community, with 3% to 4% of depressives dying by suicide today. Studies have shown that depression has considerable morbidity and mortality. This article focuses on depressed patients and their management within the emergency department. Understanding the intricacies of the interview process and identifying which patients need immediate attention are important skills for the emergency physician.

New drugs of abuse continue to emerge, including synthetic cannabinoids, synthetic cathinones, and hallucinogens. It is important to recognize their individual psychopharmacologic properties, symptoms of intoxication, and symptoms of withdrawal. Providers must be vigilant of acute medical or psychiatric complications that may arise from use of these substances. Treatment of the patient also includes recognition of any substance use disorders as well as comorbid psychiatric disorders. Although pharmacologic treatments for substance use disorder (of the drugs included in this article) are limited, there are a variety of psychotherapeutic modalities that may be of some benefit.

Difficult patients are often those who present with a mix of physical and psychiatric symptoms, and seem refractory to usual treatments or reassurance. Such patients can include those with personality disorders, those with somatization symptoms; they can come across as entitled, drug-seeking, manipulative, or simply draining to the provider. Such patients are often frequent visitors to Emergency Departments. Other reasons for difficult encounters could be rooted in provider bias or countertransference, rather than sole patient factors. Emergency providers need to have high awareness of these possibilities, and be prepared to manage such situations, otherwise workup can be sub-standard and dangerous medical mistakes can be made.

Proper treatment of the pediatric psychiatric population can be challenging. Emergency department (ED) boarding, availability of child and adolescent psychiatrists, lack of parental understanding, and inexperience working with children with special needs are just some of the obstacles the ED physician will encounter. We discuss the risk stratification and interventions necessary when dealing with children and adolescents presenting with suicidal ideation and violent behavior. In addition, we discuss the unique approaches to patients with autism spectrum disorders and attention deficit hyperactivity disorder.

With the increasing life expectancy, the geriatric population has been increasing over the past few decades. By the year 2050, it is projected to compose more than a fifth of the entire population, representing a 147% increase in this age group. There has been a steady increase in the number of medical and psychiatric disorders, and a large percentage of geriatric patients are now presenting to the emergency department with such disorders. The management of our progressively complex geriatric patient population will require an integrative team approach involving emergency medicine, psychiatry, and hospitalist medicine.

Psychiatric emergencies in pregnancy can be difficult to manage. The authors (both practicing psychiatrists and emergency clinicians) review the evaluation and treatment of common mental health diagnoses in pregnancy.

The emergent management of a traumatic injury can be an extremely intense situation. These assessments can be even more difficult when patients have an underlying psychiatric condition. After a protocoled evaluation of the traumatic injuries, the psychological manifestation of diseases can be addressed. The appropriate use of physical or chemical restraints to facilitate the work-up is paramount in the ability of the provider to protect patients and staff from agitated and traumatized patients. The emergency medicine provider should have a low threshold for including psychiatry in the treatment plans, as the long-term sequelae of these entities require specialized treatment.

The care of patients with a psychiatric emergency is fraught with ethical challenges. Applying ethical reasoning to clinical challenges may help to improve care. Emergency providers should assess decision-making capacity using 4 criteria: communication, understanding, appreciation, and reasoning. Maintaining patient confidentiality is a strong imperative for emergency physicians and should be protected unless compelling additional concerns take precedence. The goal of involuntary treatment should be to protect patients from harm that they would not be exposed to were they capable of autonomous decision making, not dangerous, or not

EMERGENCY MEDICINE
CLINICS OF NORTH AMERICA

PROGRAM OBJECTIVE

The goal of *Emergency Medicine Clinics of North America* is to keep practicing emergency medicine physicians and emergency medicine residents up to date with current clinical practice in emergency medicine by providing timely articles reviewing the state of the art in patient care.

LEARNING OBJECTIVES

Upon completion of this activity, participants will be able to:

1. Review stabilization and management techniques for agitated or psychotic patients in the emergency room.
2. Recognize psychiatric emergencies in specialized populations such as pregnant or elderly patients.
3. Discuss ethical and health policy considerations in treating mental and behavioral health emergencies.

ACCREDITATION

The Elsevier Office of Continuing Medical Education (EOCME) is accredited by the Accreditation Council for Continuing Medical Education (ACCME) to provide continuing medical education for physicians.

The EOCME designates this enduring material for a maximum of 15 *AMA PRA Category 1 Credit*(s)™. Physicians should claim only the credit commensurate with the extent of their participation in the activity.

All other health care professionals requesting continuing education credit for this enduring material will be issued a certificate of participation.

DISCLOSURE OF CONFLICTS OF INTEREST

The EOCME assesses conflict of interest with its instructors, faculty, planners, and other individuals who are in a position to control the content of CME activities. All relevant conflicts of interest that are identified are thoroughly vetted by EOCME for fair balance, scientific objectivity, and patient care recommendations. EOCME is committed to providing its learners with CME activities that promote improvements or quality in healthcare and not a specific proprietary business or a commercial interest.

The planning committee, staff, authors and editors listed below have identified no financial relationships or relationships to products or devices they or their spouse/life partner have with commercial interest related to the content of this CME activity:

Michael K. Abraham, MD, MS; Nathan Gold Allen, MD; Mohammad Shami Alzahri, MD, MSc; Sharadamani Anandan, MD; Sara Andrabi, MD; Patrick R. Aquino, MD; Bianca Asan, MD; Erin AufderHeide, MD; Rakel C. Beall, MD; Cedric Dark, MD, MPH; Elizabeth H. David, MD; Nathan Deal, MD; Araceli Flores, PhD; Anjali Fortna; Spencer Greene, MD, MS, FACEP; Thiago C. Halmer, MD, MBA; Jin Y. Han, MD; Michelle Hong, MD, PharmD; Sarathi Kalra, MD, MPH; Jeffrey Steven Khan, MD; Dick C. Kuo, MD; Indu Kumari; Benjamin Li, MD; Patrick Manley; Anu Matorin, MD; Amal Mattu, MD, FAAEM, FACEP; Nidal Moukaddam, MD, PhD; Kimberly Nordstrom, MD, JD; Ebelechukwu A. Odiari, MD; Natalie Pon, MD; Galwankar Sagar, DNB, MPH, FACEE, Diplomat. ABEM; Erin Scheckenbach; Navdeep Sekhon, MD; Asim Shah, MD; Kaylin Siever, MD; Veronica Sikka, MD, PhD, MHA, MPH, FAAEM; Andrea Gail Stolar, MD; Alexander Toledo, DO, PharmD; Mina.Tran, MD; Veronica Tucci, MD, JD; Gary M. Vilke, MD; Michael P. Wilson, MD, PhD.

UNAPPROVED/OFF-LABEL USE DISCLOSURE

The EOCME requires CME faculty to disclose to the participants:

1. When products or procedures being discussed are off-label, unlabelled, experimental, and/or investigational (not US Food and Drug Administration [FDA] approved); and
2. Any limitations on the information presented, such as data that are preliminary or that represent ongoing research, interim analyses, and/or unsupported opinions. Faculty may discuss information about pharmaceutical agents that is outside of FDA-approved labelling. This information is intended solely for CME and is not intended to promote off-label use of these medications. If you have any questions, contact the medical affairs department of the manufacturer for the most recent prescribing information.

TO ENROLL

To enroll in the *Emergency Medicine Clinics* Continuing Medical Education program, call customer service at 1-800-654-2452 or sign up online at http://www.theclinics.com/home/cme. The CME program is available to subscribers for an additional annual fee of $235 USD.

METHOD OF PARTICIPATION

In order to claim credit, participants must complete the following:

1. Complete enrolment as indicated above.
2. Read the activity.
3. Complete the CME Test and Evaluation. Participants must achieve a score of 70% on the test. All CME Tests and Evaluations must be completed online.

CME INQUIRIES/SPECIAL NEEDS

For all CME inquiries or special needs, please contact elsevierCME@elsevier.com.

Foreword
Behavioral and Psychiatric
Emergencies

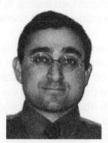

Amal Mattu, MD, FAAEM, FACEP
Consulting Editor

I'll admit that we emergency physicians (and likely many other acute care providers as well) are a strange lot. We tend to relish caring for the sickest of patients, often even those on the verge of death. We often talk about that "great case" we saw during a shift: the cardiac arrest, the crashing asthmatic with a difficult airway, the patient with sepsis or diabetic ketoacidosis with a pH of 6.9, or the patient with cardiogenic shock requiring dobutamine and norepinephrine. It's unlikely you'll ever hear one of us refer to the patient with an uncomplicated ankle sprain or gastroenteritis or migraine headache or simple pneumonia as a "great case." None of these patients tend to suffer much morbidity, and they are at low risk of mortality.

It's also unlikely that you'll ever hear an emergency physician refer to a patient with depression and failed suicide attempt, or a patient with agitated delirium from drug use, or a patient with acute psychosis as a "great case." Why not? Perhaps a major reason for this mindset is that we tend to assume that these patients have a low risk of morbidity or mortality. And perhaps another reason is that we often assume that we cannot change their course of illness. Both of these beliefs, as it turns out, are wrong, and they are likely the result of a lack of education regarding behavioral and psychiatric emergencies. Despite the fact that psychiatric illness is a rapidly increasing problem in our society and a tremendous burden on health care resources, traditional emergency medicine training still requires a relatively small amount of time be spent on this area. Continuing medical education emergency medicine conferences at the national and international level also have a paucity of sessions devoted to psychiatric and behavioral emergencies. A general lack of education leads to a lack of understanding and appreciation of the importance of this area in our practice.

We are therefore fortunate to be able to present this issue of *Emergency Medicine Clinics of North America*, in which Guest Editors Drs Kuo and Tucci have assembled an outstanding team to educate us about the latest advances and approaches to behavioral and psychiatric emergencies. Perhaps the most important of the articles

Emerg Med Clin N Am 33 (2015) xv–xvi
http://dx.doi.org/10.1016/j.emc.2015.09.002
0733-8627/15/$ – see front matter © 2015 Published by Elsevier Inc.

emed.theclinics.com

comes early in the issue and addresses the initial medical clearance of these patients. This article addresses some of the common pitfalls associated with clearance, including the frequent initial overtesting of patients that leads to increased hospital costs and emergency department (ED) lengths of stay and also addresses the pitfalls of performing cursory examinations. Readers are reminded that many patients with behavioral emergencies are suffering from underlying medical conditions that can be disastrous if not diagnosed rapidly in the ED, and that "shotgun" lab testing is inferior to the performance of a good history and physical examination when it comes to diagnosing medical illnesses.

The authors then go on to discuss the initial management and stabilization of agitated, psychotic, and delirious patients in the subsequent two articles. They address issues that go far beyond the traditional A-B-C's of emergency medicine but are equally important. Chemical and physical restraints are discussed and the laboratory workup as well. The authors also educate the readers about the challenge of distinguishing delirium from dementia and provide some nice diagnostic pearls.

Traditional psychiatric conditions are then discussed, including depression and suicidality, personality disorders, and disorders that are associated with somatic symptoms. Drug abuse and withdrawal, which are contributors to many behavioral disorders, are then addressed in a separate article. The authors provide four excellent articles that address psychiatric conditions in special populations: pediatric patients, elderly patients, pregnant patients, and trauma patients. I'd venture to guess that many acute care providers rarely give much thought to the special considerations that these latter three groups, in particular, deserve. The final articles address ethical issues in managing patients with psychiatric conditions and also health policy issues on a national level. That last article deserves special attention by anyone that is involved in public health and patient- or specialty-advocacy. The article discusses issues that we will be facing in the coming years and also the need for increased resources if we are to succeed in managing these patients properly.

The Guest Editors and authors are to be commended for their hard work. This issue of *Emergency Medicine Clinics of North America* represents an invaluable addition to the emergency medicine literature and core curriculum. Although behavioral and psychiatric emergency conditions are not generally regarded as "great cases" to deal with in the ED, readers of this issue of *Emergency Medicine Clinics of North America* will certainly develop a newfound respect for these conditions and might even develop a new level of enjoyment in managing patients that are suffering from these conditions.

Amal Mattu, MD, FAAEM, FACEP
Department of Emergency Medicine
University of Maryland
School of Medicine
Baltimore, MD, 21201, USA

E-mail address:
amalmattu@comcast.net

Preface

The Hidden Costs of Behavioral and Psychiatric Emergencies

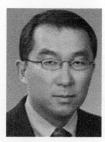
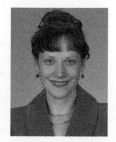

Dick C. Kuo, MD   Veronica Tucci, MD, JD
Editors

The American Psychiatric Association defines mental illness as a range of disorders characterized by the dysregulation of mood, thought, and/or behavior and defines psychiatric emergencies as acute disturbances in thought, mood, or relationships that require immediate intervention. The most pervasive mental illness is depression, and the World Health Organization (WHO) predicts that by 2030, depression, not infectious disease or cancer, will be the leading cause of disease burden globally.[1]

The statistics are indeed staggering. The Centers for Disease Control and Prevention has estimated that 25% of adults in the United States will suffer from mental illness this year and nearly 50% of adults will develop at least one mental illness during their lifetime.[2] Between 1992 and 2001, there were 53 million mental health-related Emergency Department (ED) visits in the United States. In 2002, the economic burden of mental illness in the United States was estimated to be over $300 billion dollars. By 2007, psychiatric and behavioral emergency visits doubled, and the economic burden of mental illness started to spiral even more out of control.

According to the WHO, annual spending on mental health is less than $2 per person and less than $0.25 in low-income countries. Median health expenditures per capita range from $0.20 in low-income countries to $44.84 in high-income countries.[1] Even in high-income countries like the United States, the mere pittance spent on mental illness prevention, stabilization, and treatment pales in comparison to the amount of money an average American worker spends on coffee (estimated by one study to exceed $1000 annually and over $20 per week).[3]

The limited amount of funds available for the stabilization and treatment of patients with severe mental illness had led to a marked decline in the number of beds in inpatient psychiatric facilities. Desperate and with no other place to go, patients with psychiatric emergencies are turning in droves to their local EDs.

This issue of *Emergency Medicine Clinics of North America* is designed to aid emergency physicians in the management of acute exacerbations of mental illness. To that

Emerg Med Clin N Am 33 (2015) xvii–xviii
http://dx.doi.org/10.1016/j.emc.2015.09.001
0733-8627/15/$ – see front matter © 2015 Published by Elsevier Inc.

emed.theclinics.com

end, we have provided comprehensive and up-to-date literature reviews on several high-impact topics in the field of behavioral emergencies, including navigating the medical clearance process, stabilizing the acutely agitated or psychotic patient, differentiating etiologies of altered mental status, identifying and managing depressed and suicidal patients, strategies for successfully patients with personality and somatoform disorders, addressing specific concerns of special populations, including pediatric, geriatric, pregnant, and trauma patients.

Dick C. Kuo, MD
Section of Emergency Medicine
Department of Medicine
Baylor College of Medicine
1504 Taub Loop
Emergency Center Academic Offices
1EC 61 002
Houston, TX 77030, USA

Veronica Tucci, MD, JD
Section of Emergency Medicine
Department of Medicine
Baylor College of Medicine
1504 Taub Loop
Houston, TX 77030, USA

E-mail addresses:
dckuo@bcm.edu (D.C. Kuo)
vtuccimd@gmail.com (V. Tucci)

REFERENCES

1. Available at: http://apps.who.int/gb/ebwha/pdf_files/EB130/B130_9-en.pdf. Accessed August 10, 2015.
2. Available at: http://www.cdc.gov/mentalhealthsurveillance/. Accessed August 10, 2015.
3. Available at: http://consumerist.com/2012/01/20/most-american-workers-spend-more-than-1000year-on-coffee/. Accessed August 10, 2015.

Down the Rabbit Hole

Emergency Department Medical Clearance of Patients with Psychiatric or Behavioral Emergencies

Veronica Tucci, MD, JD[a],*, Kaylin Siever, MD[a], Anu Matorin, MD[b],
Nidal Moukaddam, MD, PhD[b]

KEYWORDS

- Medical clearance • Medical screening • Medical stability
- Psychiatric and behavioral emergencies

KEY POINTS

- Patients with primary mental health complaints comprise a substantial proportion of all emergency department visits.
- The medical clearance process for patients with behavioral and psychiatric emergencies consists of several elements, including medically stabilizing patients and meeting criteria for various inpatient psychiatric hospitals with limited medical resources.
- There are no uniformly accepted interdisciplinary guidelines or algorithms that constitute medical clearance between psychiatry and emergency medicine.
- The breadth of ancillary testing, including laboratory examinations and radiographic evaluations, is often hotly debated among EPs, emergency psychiatrists, and inpatient psychiatry teams.

INTRODUCTION

"But I don't want to go among mad people," Alice remarked.
"Oh, you can't help that," said the Cat: "we're all mad here. I'm mad. You're mad."
"How do you know I'm mad?" said Alice.
"You must be," said the Cat, "or you wouldn't have come here."
—Lewis Carroll, Alice in Wonderland

Disclosure: The authors have nothing to disclose.
[a] Section of Emergency Medicine, Baylor College of Medicine, 1504 Taub Loop, Houston, TX 77030, USA; [b] Menninger Department of Psychiatry and Behavioral Sciences, Baylor College of Medicine, 1502 Taub Loop, NPC Building 2nd Floor, Houston, TX 77030, USA
* Corresponding author.
E-mail addresses: Tucci@bcm.edu; vtuccimd@gmail.com

Emerg Med Clin N Am 33 (2015) 721–737
http://dx.doi.org/10.1016/j.emc.2015.07.002   emed.theclinics.com

Although the Cheshire cat was describing Wonderland to Alice, his words could have just as easily been spoken by a triage nurse during a busy overnight shift in an urban emergency department (ED). Imagine an ambulance bay and waiting room teeming with intoxicated, agitated, and psychotic patients. Surely, this dark and depressing image must be the backdrop of an urban legend, twisted fairy tale, or some cheesy made-for-TV medical drama. Then again, maybe it is merely the hallucination of some emergency staffer, high on monster drinks. When being outflanked at every turn by the inebriated and psychotic, in the words of Alice, would it really be mad of the emergency physicians (EPs) and emergency psychiatrists "to pray for better hallucinations?"

The ED serves as both the lifeline and the gateway to psychiatric care for millions of patients suffering from acute behavioral or psychiatric emergencies.[1] The American Psychiatric Association (APA) defines psychiatric emergencies as situations involving acute disturbances or alterations in "thought, mood, or social relationships that require immediate intervention as defined by patient, family or social unit."[2,3]

These thought and mood disturbances can manifest in a myriad of ways and with varying degrees of severity. Patients may complain of anxiety or depression, experience personality changes, hallucinations, or delusions or show violent, aggressive, or self-injurious behavior. Psychiatric chief complaints already represent a staggering 6% of all adult ED visits and 7% of all pediatric ED visits, with the number increasing annually.[4,5] Like the Queen of Hearts, when confronted with the unique challenges and complexity inherent in the care of these patients, the overwhelmed EP may be tempted to yell, "Off with their heads," thereby removing a large burden on the system and decompressing the triage area. However, as medical providers used to operating as a safety net for the most vulnerable members of our society, EPs cannot and will not so callously abandon their charges.

In a sense, the EP is the patient's guide through Wonderland, ushering them safely from the ED into the hands of qualified psychiatric providers. The first and most important step of this process is to provide the medical clearance necessary for inpatient psychiatric admission.

Although there is no uniformly accepted definition of or interdisciplinary standard for medical clearance, EPs are generally charged with determining whether the patient's psychiatric or behavioral emergency is the result of organic/functional or psychological conditions. When symptoms have a medical cause, inpatient psychiatric hospitalization is obviated. Psychiatric patients already have long ED stays, high rates of admission, readmission, and return visits, and high medical costs; it is a challenge to provide an accurate and complete medical assessment without ordering tests that unnecessarily compound the problem.[6,7] In this article, the controversies behind the medical clearance process are discussed and strategies for providing medical clearance in a cost-conscious manner are discussed.

Impact of Psychiatric Disease on the Emergency System

Adult patients with psychiatric and behavioral emergencies accounted for more than 53 million ED visits from 1992 to 2001 in the United States.[4] More recent data have shown an alarming trend of increasing ED visits for primary mental health complaints. For example, the Centers for Disease Control reported that during 2010 to 2011, approximately 468,000 ED visits were made by patients with bipolar disorder.[8]

In Harris County (where the authors work primarily), an estimated 108,480 children and 140,000 adults have a severe mental illness warranting treatment. With only 800 inpatient beds available in a population that requires an estimated 2000 beds, more than 650 patients are seen, stabilized and treated in the ED of Ben Taub General

Hospital alone each month. Approximately two-thirds of patients seen in the ED are discharged home. Twenty-two percent are transferred to an inpatient psychiatric facility, and 9% are admitted overnight to the ED locked psychiatric unit. The average length of stay for patients with psychiatric complaints who are medically cleared and discharged home after being evaluated by emergency psychiatry in the ED is 14.6 hours; for those who are medically cleared and admitted to the ED locked unit, it is 18.7 hours; and for those who are transferred/admitted to and inpatient facility, it is 29.5 hours (Matorin and Shah, unpublished, 2014). In this type of psychiatric emergency service (PES) model, there is around-the-clock staffing with mental health professionals; patients are not only treated but can often be stabilized, which can decrease inpatient admissions.[9]

Similarly, data from 2008 to 2010 in North Carolina showed that although the annual number of ED visits increased by 5.1%, the number of ED visits for mental health–related complaints increased by 17.7%, (from 347,806 to 409,276).[10]

As the only medical care available 24 hours a day, 7 days a week, and 365 days a year, EPs are often tasked with evaluating, stabilizing, and treating patients with acute psychiatric conditions. This early intervention and care have been shown to decrease morbidity and mortality.[11,12] An appropriate and accurate medical clearance process is imperative for decreasing time to disposition and cost as well as identifying medical issues that may be causing or exacerbating the patient's presentation or that may need to be treated (or are inappropriate to treat) in an inpatient psychiatric setting.[13]

ED directors report significant limitations in available resources to care for patients with behavioral and psychiatric complaints. Those surveyed expressed a need for solutions to nonemergent mental health problems presenting to the ED, including improved access to mental health personnel in ED evaluations, outpatient community mental health resources, and mechanisms for patient referrals.[14] Interdisciplinary collaboration between EPs and psychiatrists is essential.

The strained mental health system, coupled with a lack of both outpatient and inpatient resources, necessitates that the initial evaluation and management of these patients are performed in the ED. High patient volume, staff attitudes, issues with the medical clearance process, and inappropriate assessment of agitation level can all negatively affect the care of psychiatric patients.[15]

Emergency boarding (an emerging phenomenon that refers to when patients stay in the ED while waiting for inpatient psychiatric admission) has also complicated the medical clearance process. Boarded patients not only have a longer length of stay but their conditions are often not treated while awaiting inpatient hospitalization.[13] One study found that the overall mean length of stay was 11.5 hours.

Medical complications and evolving clinical pictures in this patient population sometimes call for continued emergency medicine services. The need for hospitalization, restraint use, and completion of diagnostic imaging had the greatest effect on postassessment boarding time, whereas the presence of alcohol and toxicology screening led to delays earlier in the stay.[6]

Pediatric Patients with Psychiatric Complaints

These challenges of providing medical clearance to individuals with mental health issues are not limited to the adult population. The pediatric portion of this population is increasing, and the ED often provides a safety net.[15] Between 1993 and 1999, there were an average of 434,000 ED pediatric mental health visits, and this population accounted for 1.6% of all ED visits for this age group. Although a study found that this number increased during those years, there was no increase in the 2 patient categories that are mandatorily seen in EDs: psychosis and suicide attempt.[16] This finding suggested that the overall increase was attributed to nonurgent complaints that could be managed in the outpatient setting.[16] These results again reflect the overall strain on and lack of resources in the outpatient mental health setting.

In 2011, the American Academy of Pediatrics Committee on Pediatric Emergency Medicine published a technical report on pediatric mental health emergencies in the emergency setting. The committee identified challenges including inpatient bed shortages, insurance issues, and a lack of pediatric trained mental health specialists. The committee suggested that this situation could ideally be addressed by restructuring the outpatient setting, local level planning, and community resources, strengthening mental health support networks, and educating primary care providers. A 3-pronged approach was devised, consisting of education, research, and advocacy for improvement of accurate and timely ED management of these patients. Other suggestions included strategies to enlist the family and primary care providers as partners to provide basic psychiatric care and access to the mental health system.[15]

Medical Clearance Definition and Background

Inpatient psychiatric facilities generally require emergency providers to perform a medical evaluation of patients presenting to the ED with psychiatric complaints before those patients are referred or transferred to the psychiatric facility. The term for this process is medical clearance.

However, this term is imprecise and often misunderstood.[17–19] Several issues have been proposed with the term medical clearance. One study showed that "medically clear" was documented in 80% of patients' charts in which medical diseases should have been identified.[19] Adding to this confusion is the lack of consensus between psychiatrists and EP about what medical clearance should entail.[20] Some providers require medically clear patients to have no medical illness or comorbid conditions. Other providers suggest that medically clear patients can have a coexisting medical illness if these illnesses are not believed to be the cause of the current psychiatric symptoms (eg, a urinary tract infection in an otherwise healthy young adult). Other providers permit patients to be medically cleared even when a medical illness may have caused or contributed to the patient's symptoms but when treatment is no longer needed (eg, history of hypertensive encephalopathy in a patient who is now normotensive).[18,20]

The lifespan of individuals with mental illness is approximately 8 years shorter than the lifespan of individuals in the general population.[21] Moreover, patients with psychiatric illness have a higher incidence of medical conditions as well as a greater risk of injury.[22–24] Often, patients are termed medically clear when they have medical problems that needed to be addressed or need continued treatment or management. Some providers believe that the term medical assessment more accurately reflects the needs of this population and that the medical clearance process should be replaced by a more thorough discharge note with specific recommendations for the management of any underlying medical conditions.[19] This note should include medical diagnoses and recommendations for management and follow-up, instructions, and instructions for medication administration.[19]

Regardless of the term used, medical evaluation is needed for possible underlying organic causes that may cause, or exacerbate, the patient's presenting behavioral symptoms. It is also important to identify factors that may require further or ongoing treatment or that may affect treatment decisions and medication choices (eg, a positive pregnancy test). Other considerations include the capability of the receiving psychiatry facility to accommodate medical needs (eg, indwelling Foley catheters) and functional requirements of those facilities.[18]

In 2006, the American College of Emergency Physicians (ACEP) published a clinical policy addressing medical clearance in *Annals of Emergency Medicine*. This policy is summarized in **Box 1**.

The APA guideline recommendations for the evaluation of the emergency psychiatric patient are outlined in **Box 2**.[25]

Psychiatric providers place a higher importance on the results of urine drug screens and alcohol levels because patients cannot be diagnosed with de novo psychiatric diagnoses while under the influence of mood-altering and mind-altering substances. Acute alcohol/drug intoxication and withdrawal can mimic psychological conditions so the patient can be diagnosed only when sober.[26]

The ACEP and APA guidelines for medical clearance/evaluation place different values on substance abuse and toxicology screening in the ED.[26,27] Lack of interdisciplinary agreement can lead to the adoption of arbitrary exclusionary criteria at inpatient facilities and delay patient transfer.

CLINICAL EVALUATION
Approach to the Patient with Psychiatric Complaints

Overall, the approach to patients presenting with behavioral complaints should be the same as the approach to those with general medical conditions. The patient's clinical findings should guide diagnostic testing, including laboratory tests, imaging, consultations, and interventions.[1] The approach to the psychiatric patient in the emergency room begins with the ABCs (airway, breathing, circulation), and addressing any life-threatening concerns. Because patients presenting with psychiatric complaints are often at risk for traumatic injury (either self-inflicted or from third parties) or other life-threatening medical conditions requiring immediate resuscitation (eg, cardiopulmonary collapse from an overdose of medication), we recommend that physicians

---

Box 1
Summary of ACEP medical clearance guidelines

Level B recommendations

1. In adult ED patients with primary psychiatric complaints, diagnostic evaluation should be directed by the history and physical examination.

2. Routine laboratory testing of all patients is of low yield and need not be performed as part of the ED assessment.

Level C recommendations regarding UDS

1. Routine urine toxicologic screens for drugs of abuse in alert, awake, cooperative patients do not affect ED management and need not be performed as part of the ED assessment.

2. Urine toxicologic screens for drugs of abuse obtained in the ED for the use of the receiving psychiatric facility or service should not delay patient evaluation or transfer.

Level C recommendations regarding EtOH

1. The patient's cognitive abilities, rather than a specific blood alcohol level, should be the basis on which clinicians begin the psychiatric assessment.

2. Consider using a period of observation to determine if psychiatric symptoms resolve as the episode of intoxication resolves.

Data from Lukens TW, Wolf SJ, Edlow JA, et al. Clinical policy: critical issues in the diagnosis and management of the adult psychiatric patient in the emergency department. Ann Emergency Med 2006;47:79–99.

Box 2
Elements/domains of a clinical psychiatric evaluation

History of present illness

Psychiatric history

History of alcohol and substance use

General medical history

Developmental, psychosocial, and sociocultural history

Occupational and military history

Legal history

Family history

Review of systems

Physical examination

Mental status examination

Functional assessment

Laboratory assessment including urine drug screens

Provisional diagnosis most likely responsible for presentation

Data from American Psychiatric Association. American Psychiatric Association practice guidelines for the treatment of psychiatric disorders: compendium 2006. Arlington (VA): American Psychiatric Publication; 2006; and American Psychiatric Association Steering Committee on Practice Guidelines. Psychiatric evaluation of adults, a quick reference guide. Arlington (VA): American Psychiatric Association Practice Guidelines; 2006. p. 1–18.

---

performing the medical clearance examination should follow an algorithm similar to that used in advanced trauma life support and advanced cardiopulmonary life support courses.[28,29] This algorithm is presented in **Fig. 1**.

Next, a thorough history and physical examination should seek to identify if there is an organic or psychiatric cause to the symptoms as well as whether or not the patient's behavior complaint has led to a behavior that poses a medical threat that needs to be addressed.[28–30] The distinction of functional versus organic cause is imperative, because the latter is often reversible, and failure to diagnose an organic cause may be catastrophic. Examples of this are bacterial meningitis or a subdural hematoma.[29,30] Physicians should have a low threshold to evaluate for self-injurious behavior.[29] Although a previous psychiatric history is important to identify, it should not lead to the assumption that the patient's current symptoms do not have an organic cause.

Several studies have stressed the importance of a thorough evaluation for identifying an underlying medical cause. A study performed in 1978 of 658 consecutive psychiatric outpatients found an incidence of 9.1% of medical disorders presenting as

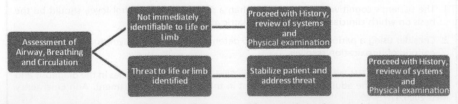

Fig. 1. Assessment and stabilization of threat to life or limb in the psychiatric patient.

psychiatric complaints. Visual hallucinations were a strong indicator of this situation. Most frequently, the cause was infection, pulmonary, thyroid dysfunction, diabetes, hematopoietic, hepatic, and central nervous system (CNS) disease.[31,32] Another study performed in the PES of the Royal Ottowa Hospital investigated patients with psychiatric complaints who had physical disorders requiring immediate treatment or investigation.[33] The investigators found this group to comprise 7% of the patient population. Those with physical problems tended to be older than 60 years and were diagnosed with alcoholic or chronic organic brain syndrome.[33]

History

The history starts by obtaining a detailed description of recent symptoms and current changes in behavior of the patient. Although this history may be provided by the patient, an attempt should be made to obtain collateral information. EPs should try to obtain a history from as many ancillary sources as possible (eg, family, emergency medical services, police). These additional sources can provide a baseline for the patient's symptoms and confirm the story (especially if the patient's mental capacity is impaired or not known). This information is also helpful if the patient is unable or unwilling to provide a history. Sudden changes in behavior from a previously normal patient or definite deterioration of those with an underlying disorder should prompt a search for underlying organic cause.[1,34]

MEDICAL PROBLEMS PRESENTING AS PSYCHIATRIC COMPLAINTS

Recorded history is rife with examples of vague and unusual symptoms that physicians attributed to psychiatric conditions but were later shown to be true, organic disease. One of the most famous examples is King George III, whose "insanity" was caused by porphyria.[35] EPs must be cognizant of these psychiatric mimics and wherever possible ferret out any medical explanations for apparent psychiatric conditions.[29] Examples are provided in **Box 3**.

The history, evaluation, and physical examination should be aimed at maximizing the chance of identifying the patients who fall into this category, minimizing the use of unnecessary testing. A complete and accurate history and physical examination help to accomplish this.

There are several historical features, summarized in **Table 1**, that make an organic diagnosis more likely.[34,36,38] New psychiatric complaints should be assumed to be medical until proved otherwise.[34]

Patients with no previous history of psychiatric diagnoses have a greater likelihood of an underlying medical disorder causing their presentation and require an evaluation. This finding was shown in a study of 100 consecutive patients with new psychiatric symptoms over a 9-month period. Each received a history and physical examination, complete blood count (CBC), Sequential Multiple Analysis-7, prothrombin time, calcium, oxygen saturation, creatine phosphokinase if there was possible myoglobinuria, alcohol level, urine drug screen, computed tomography scan of the patient's head, and a lumbar puncture if febrile. The investigators found that 63 of 100 patients had an organic cause of their symptoms. The medical history was significant in 27 of these patients, and physical examination was significant in 6. The investigators concluded that most alert, adult patients with new psychiatric symptoms have an organic cause for their condition.[39]

Symptoms of current or recent infections should be evaluated if present because delirium may present an acute psychiatric disorder.[36,38] The distinction between psychiatric disease and delirium is important because delirium is associated with a

> **Box 3**
> **Organic conditions masquerading as psychiatric disease**
>
> Autoimmune disorders: systemic lupus erythematosus, myasthenia gravis, multiple sclerosis
>
> CNS disease: space-occupying lesions
>
> Drug and medication disorders/side effects: cocaine abuse/intoxication, synthetic cannabis use
>
> Electrolyte abnormalities: hypercalcemia
>
> Endocrine disorders: including hyperthyroidism, hypothyroidism/myxedema coma, Addison disease, insulinoma, panhypopituitarism, DKA, pheochromocytoma
>
> Environmental disorders: hypothermia
>
> Hematologic disorders: thrombotic thrombocytopenic purpura
>
> Hereditary metabolic disorders: Wilson disease, urea cycle disorders, Niemann-Pick type C, porphyria, Tay-Sachs
>
> Infectious disorders: neurosyphilis, sepsis, HIV, cerebral malaria, neurocysticercosis, herpes encephalitis
>
> Metabolic disorders: hepatic encephalopathy, uremia, paraneoplastic syndromes
>
> Nutritional deficiencies: vitamin B_{12}
>
> Poisonings: botulism, heavy metals, carbon monoxide
>
> Withdrawal syndromes: delirium tremens, Wernicke-Korsakoff

significant increase in mortality.[40] A thorough discussion of these conditions is beyond the scope of this article and can be found elsewhere in this issue. Similarly, physicians should inquire about recent medication changes as well as medication compliance/adherence and the use of mood-altering substances. An evaluation of the patient's mental status is an important component of the physical examination.[41]

Patients reporting any of the historical features noted in **Table 1** should receive further workup and focused testing.

> **Table 1**
> **Comparison of historical features distinguishing organic causes of psychiatric complaints from true psychological or functional disease**
>
> | Organic | Psychiatric |
> |---|---|
> | Age <12 y or >40 y without previous psychiatric diagnosis | Previous psychiatric diagnosis >12 y and <40 y |
> | Sudden onset of symptoms | Gradual development of symptoms |
> | Visual or tactile hallucinations | Auditory hallucinations |
> | History of substance abuse | No recent ingestions of mind-altering substances or toxins |
> | New medications (including over-the-counter and herbal medications) | No new medications |
> | Seizure | No seizures |
> | No family history of psychiatric disorders | Significant family history (including first-degree relatives) of psychiatric disorders |
>
> Data from Refs.[1,28,29,34,36,37]

Medical comorbidities and complaints must be evaluated thoroughly, because these cannot only cause or exacerbate psychiatric symptoms but have treatment implications for both acute and chronic medical disorders if the patient is admitted to an inpatient psychiatric facility.

All acute medical conditions should be addressed and stabilized before patient transfer to an inpatient psychiatric facility. EPs should make recommendations to ensure symptom resolution (eg, prescription for doxycycline to treat acute pelvic inflammatory disease) and outpatient medical follow-up as necessary.

EPs should also remember that medical conditions can exacerbate preexisting psychiatric disorders and aggressively manage comorbid medical conditions. A study in 2004[42] investigated medical comorbidity in individuals with serious mental illness who were receiving community-based psychiatric treatment. Two hundred outpatients with diagnoses of schizophrenia or affective disorders were evaluated, and their responses were matched to controls. In the final analysis, both groups had greater odds of having medical comorbidities compared with controls, including respiratory illness, diabetes, and liver disorders.

Review of Systems

The review of symptoms may also help to identify any underlying medical cause, and history should be tailored to exploring the positive findings.[1] For example, weight gain and cold intolerance might lead to evaluation for underlying thyroid disorder. A history of high-risk sexual behavior, lymphadenopathy, weight loss, and upper respiratory tract symptoms may prompt screening for human immunodeficiency virus (HIV). Patients with HIV can present with behavioral disturbances caused by CNS lesions or infections.

Physical Examination

The aim of the physical examination is to identify medical disorders that may cause or exacerbate the underlying condition or diagnoses that may need treatment or special care or that cannot be managed in an inpatient psychiatric setting.[1] In general, the physical examination should be dictated by the individual patient presentation and complaints, and known medical comorbidities.

First, physicians must obtain a full set of vital signs and address any abnormalities.[1] It may be difficult to initially obtain vital signs in an agitated or hostile patient, but they should be obtained as soon as possible and rechecked before discharge. Abnormal vital signs are often the harbinger of serious underlying disease.[34]

Patients with limited histories (eg, those with altered mental status or who are intoxicated) or who have self-inflicted injuries should have a full physical examination.[29] All patients should be evaluated for trauma or symptoms suggestive of an ingestion or toxidrome. Otherwise, the depth of the physical examination in the ED depends on the complaints.[29] **Table 2** summarizes physical examination features that may help the EP differentiate organic from psychiatric disease.

All patients should also have a focused, brief, and systematic mental status examination to differentiate functional, organic, and cognitive disorders.[1,41,43] Common mental status examination include the mini-mental status examination, the brief mental status examination and quick confusion scale. These tools generally focus on 7 major areas: affect, attention, language, orientation, memory, visual-spatial ability, and conceptualization.[30] Incorporating elements of the physical and psychiatric examinations, EPs can conduct a significant portion of these examinations by observing and interacting with the patient.[1,29,41,44]

Table 2
Comparison of physical examination features distinguishing organic causes of psychiatric complaints from true psychological or functional disease

Organic	Psychiatric
Abnormal vital signs	Normal vital signs
Fluctuating level of consciousness	Consistent level of consciousness
Focal neurologic findings	Normal neurologic examination
Evidence of trauma (eg, raccoon eyes, Battle sign)	No evidence of trauma
Abnormal dermatologic manifestations (eg, rashes, purpura, jaundice, uremic frost)	No skin changes
Abnormal mini-mental examination or quick confusion scale	Normal mini-mental or quick confusion scale examination

Data from Refs.[1,34,41]

Deficiencies in the Initial Assessment

Several studies have reported concern over the thoroughness of the history and physical examination obtained in the ED.

An inadequate assessment can lead to missed diagnoses and increased dependence on ancillary testing or imaging, as well as safety concerns for patients with missed medical diagnoses admitted to psychiatric facilities with limited capabilities to diagnose or manage them.

A retrospective chart review of adult patients who presented over 1 year with the diagnosis of schizophrenia was analyzed for 17 quantitative and qualitative variables. Overall, the findings suggested that complete physical examinations were regularly lacking. Complete vital signs were documented in only 52% of cases, and 6% of patients had no vital signs ever recorded. Older patients were more likely to receive full examinations.[45] Another study investigated unrecognized medical emergencies admitted to psychiatric units and attempted to determine the cause of the missed diagnosis. In 34% of cases, severe alcohol or drug intoxication was missed. A total of 12.5% of cases of withdrawal or delirium tremens were missed, and 12.5% of prescription drug overdoses were not identified. Other missed diagnoses included uremia, hepatic encephalopathy, diabetic ketoacidosis (DKA), hypoglycemia, Wernicke encephalopathy, lithium toxicity, hyperthyroidism, anticonvulsant toxicity encephalitis, pneumonia, sepsis, urinary tract infection, neurosyphilis, cerebrovascular accident, congestive heart failure, subdural hematoma, and neuroleptic malignant syndrome.[46] Several deficiencies in evaluations were noted, and in none of these patients was an appropriate mental status examination performed. A total of 43.8% had inadequate physical examinations, and 34.4% failed to obtain an available history. The investigators also cited that 34.3% failed to obtain appropriate laboratory studies.[46]

Abnormal vital signs were not addressed in almost 8% of patients.[46] Vital signs are vital and must be addressed in performing the medical clearance or medical assessment for patients with psychiatric complaints, because they are often the harbinger of more serious organic causes of psychiatric complaints or comorbid conditions that may alter the level of treatment necessary for these patients.

In 1990, deficiencies in the physical examinations performed in the ED on medically cleared patients found the following frequency with which various portions of the history and physical examination were performed: vital signs (68%), general appearance (36%), complete history of present illness (33%), heart (64%), HEENT (head, eyes, ears, nose, and throat) (63%), lungs (60%), abdomen (26%), extremities (17%), skin (4%), and musculoskeletal (1%). A total of 8% of cases had no physical examination performed.[47] Laboratory tests were ordered in 8% of patients. The investigators noted that significant medical findings were present in 12% of these patients. However, most of these were increased blood sugar levels and blood pressure, none of which required medical admission.[47]

A study performed in 1994[19] investigated 298 ED patients with psychiatric complaints, all admitted voluntarily to a psychiatric unit. Multiple deficiencies in the physical examination were found. This finding included no mental status examination in 56% of patients. Twelve of these patients required acute medical treatment in 24 hours; the investigators concluded that the ED history and physical examination should have identified an acute process in 83% of patients. Patients older than 55 years had a 4 times greater likelihood of a missed diagnosis.[25] Similarly, in a study of 1340 patients admitted to a Veterans Affairs hospital psychiatric unit and 613 to a public hospital psychiatric unit from 2001 to 2007,[48] 2.8% of records reviewed had a medical disorder that was determined to have caused their symptoms. Compared with patients in medical units, these patients who were admitted to psychiatric units had lower rates of completion of medical histories, physical examinations, cognitive assessments, indicated laboratory or radiologic studies, and treatment of abnormal vital signs.

A group set out to determine if a tool using historical and physical examination data could screen patients with psychiatric complaints for serious organic causes. If criteria for their screening tool were met, they were transferred without further laboratory or imaging studies. The investigators then reviewed charts of the ED and crisis center to determine if any of the patients required further medical treatment or admission rather than psychiatric admission. Six patients were sent back to the ED, and after further testing, none required more than an outpatient prescription. The investigators concluded that the screening tool was useful to determine if these patients needed further medical evaluation beyond history and physical examination.[49]

In 1981 an article on diagnostic errors in the evaluation of behavior disorders was published in the Journal of the American Medical Association. The investigators found that in 215 patients referred to a specialized medical-psychiatric inpatient unit, thorough neuropsychiatric evaluation resulted in a therapeutically important alteration of the referring diagnosis in 41%. Of patients referred for a tentative diagnosis of dementia, 63% were found to have treatable conditions. The investigators found that these erroneous diagnoses were provided roughly equally by psychiatric and medical practitioners; they suggested that ideally evaluation would be performed by neurologists or psychiatrists with specialty expertise in neuropsychiatric evaluation.[50]

One study found that patients younger than 55 years had a greater chance of a missed medical diagnosis, which may be counterintuitive, because this population has a lower rate of medical comorbidities. The investigators hypothesized that this situation was caused by erroneous assumptions made by the medical practitioners that patients in this group were healthier and, as a result, did not need as comprehensive a medical evaluation as older populations.[19]

Box 4 summarizes common deficiencies in the initial assessment.

Box 4
Pitfalls in the medical clearance process

Incomplete history, including failure to obtain ancillary information

Incomplete physical examination (eg, failure to perform a thorough neurologic or mental status examination)

Ignoring vital sign abnormalities

Missing threats to life or limb (eg, delirium)

Premature closure and not revisiting diagnosis of primary psychiatric condition

Indiscriminate laboratory and radiographic testing

LABORATORY AND ANCILLARY TESTING
Importance and Usefulness

Laboratory testing for the purpose of medical clearance is controversial. As noted earlier, ACEP policy indicates that testing (if any) should be guided by the patient's presentation, history, and physical examination finding, whereas the APA includes urine drug and alcohol screens. Uniform order sets are costly and have limited usefulness. Although several studies have investigated the optimal evaluation of these patients, there is no interdisciplinary consensus and the extent of testing, and it continues to be a source of debate.

In 1 retrospective, consecutive chart review,[51] 38% of patients had isolated psychiatric complaints, documented psychiatric histories, and normal physical examinations, including vital signs. In this cohort, none had positive screening or laboratory results. The remaining 62% of patients in the study presented with a medical complaint (eg, chest pain) or past medical histories that required evaluation, and the initial complaint was found to correlate directly with the need for ancillary testing for medical clearance.[51] The investigators concluded that a patient who denied current medical problems and who presented with a primary psychiatric complaint, documented psychiatric history, stable vital signs, and normal physical examination findings could be referred for psychiatric evaluation without additional testing.[51]

A similar retrospective observational analysis of 345 psychiatric patients looked at the sensitivities of the history, physical examination, vital signs, CBC, and comprehensive metabolic panel for identifying medical problems. In this study, most medical problems and substance abuse were identified by abnormal vital signs and history and physical examination.[52] The investigators concluded that universal laboratory and toxicologic screening of all patients with psychiatric complaints was low yield.[52]

In 2004, in light of conflicting data available on the merits of different screening procedures for medical clearance, a systematic review was performed, including 12 studies that reported specific yields of various screening procedures.[44] Results indicated that medical history, physical examination, review of systems, and tests for orientation had relatively high yield for detecting active medical problems and routine testing was low yield.[44] However, there were 4 groups that were at higher risk: the elderly, substance users, patients with no previous psychiatric history, and patients with preexisting medical disorders or concurrent medical complaints.[44]

Fig. 2 is an algorithm that we have developed to assist providers in determining whether a patient requires additional laboratory or radiographic testing before being medically cleared.

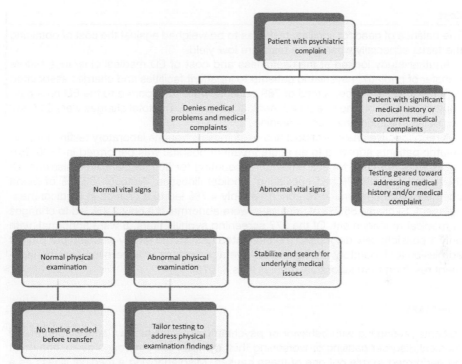

Fig. 2. Algorithm for determining the need for ancillary testing in patients presenting with psychiatric chief complaints.

Ancillary Testing in Pediatric Patients

Findings have been similar in pediatric populations. A 2014 retrospective chart review of consecutive pediatric patients in 2009 to 2010 assessed history, physical examination, and laboratory screening tests, as well as length of stay by laboratory test performed. The investigators identified 1088 visits resulting in 13,725 laboratory tests. A total of 871 visits had laboratory tests performed. Of these visits, 0.8% were associated with disposition changes, and 5.7% resulted in management changes. Twenty-five patients with noncontributory history and physical examination results had management changes (all nonurgent). Only 1 patient with a noncontributory history and physical examination had a disposition-changing laboratory result, and this was a positive urine pregnancy test. Patients with screening tests had a significantly longer length or stay. No patient was found to have an organic cause to their symptoms according to only screening tests.[53]

In 2011, a separate study assessed the usefulness and financial implications of routine laboratory screening of child and adolescent psychiatric patients after admission. Although 97.2% of all patients who received a screening laboratory test had at least 1 abnormal finding, only 4 test results (<0.5%) affected the patient's psychiatric treatment plan or required immediate medical attention. The investigators noted an average cost per patient of $33 to $122, which translated to an average yearly direct cost of $38,000.[54]

Diagnostic testing should be reserved for those with suspicious findings on clinical examination, high-risk populations, and those should be geared toward answering specific questions (see **Fig. 1**).

Cost

The balance of need for ancillary tests has to be weighed against the cost of obtaining the tests, especially when those tests are low yield.

Another study looked at the usefulness and cost of ED medical clearance before transfer of pediatric psychiatric patients to inpatient facilities and charges associated with medical clearance. A total of 789 patients were transported to the ED on a psychiatric hold, 72 of whom required medical screening. The total charges were $17,240 per patient requiring medical screening.[55]

A retrospective analysis of cost and usefulness of routine laboratory testing for psychiatric patients admitted to an acute inpatient hospital was performed in 1990. Records were obtained for 252 patients, accounting for 305 sequential admissions. Of these patients, 49.6% had coexisting medical illnesses. Although 86.2% of blood chemistry examinations were abnormal, only 4.7% led to a change in medical management. Similarly, 85.3% of urinalyses were abnormal but only 2.2% led to changes in medical management. Of the 277 screening syphilis titers, 5 were abnormal, with only 1 possibly new diagnosis. The estimated cost to the facility was $65 per patient admission for laboratory testing and the average cost per change in medical management resulting from laboratory studies was $1070.[56]

SUMMARY

Patients presenting with behavior or psychiatric complaints may have an underlying medical disorder causing or worsening their symptoms. A thorough evaluation must be performed to rule out one of these causes. Misdiagnosing a medical illness as a psychiatric one can lead to increased morbidity and mortality. A thorough history and physical examination, including mental status, is important to identify these causes and guide further testing. However, often, important portions of this process are missing or are not performed. Laboratory and ancillary testing should be guided by what is indicated based on clinical assessment, but for this to be effective, a complete clinical assessment must be performed. There are certain patient populations and signs and symptoms that have a higher association with organic causes of behavioral complaints, and the presence or absence of these entities should be explored during the initial assessment. Many medical problems can present with or exacerbate psychiatric symptoms, and a careful and thorough medical assessment is imperative for identifying these.

The complexity of the medical clearance and assessment process may make EPs and emergency psychiatrists ask "Have I gone mad?" Perhaps so; however, in the words of Lewis Carroll, "the best people usually are."

REFERENCES

1. Tintinalli JE, Stapczynski JS. Tintinalli's emergency medicine: a comprehensive study guide. New York: McGraw-Hill; 2011.
2. Hall RC, Gardner ER, Popkin MK, et al. Unrecognized physical illness prompting psychiatric admission: a prospective study. Am J Psychiatry 1981;138:629–35.
3. Allen MH, Forster P, Zealberg J, et al. APA task force on psychiatric emergency services: report and recommendations regarding psychiatric emergency and crisis services. Arlington (VA): American Psychiatric Association; 2002. p. 1–100.
4. Larkin GH, Claassen CA, Emond JA, et al. Trends in US emergency department visits for mental health conditions, 1992 to 2001. Psychiatr Serv 2005;56:671–7.

5. Simon AE, Schoendorf KC. Emergency department visits for mental health conditions among US children, 2001-2011. Clin Pediatr 2014;53:1359–66.
6. Weiss AP, Chang G, Rauch SL, et al. Patient- and practice- related determinants of emergency department length of stay for patients with psychiatric illness. Ann Emerg Med 2012;60:162–71.e5.
7. Smith MW, Stocks C, Santora PB. Hospital readmission rates and emergency department visits for mental health and substance abuse conditions. Community Ment Health J 2015;51:190–7.
8. Cherry DK, McCraig LF. Average annual rate of emergency department visits for bipolar disorder among persons aged > 15 years by age group–national hospital ambulatory medical care survey, United States, 2010-2011. Available at: www.cdc.gov/mmwr/preview/mmwrhtml/mm6349a12.htm.
9. Zeller SL. Treatment of psychiatric patients in emergency settings. Prim Psychiatry 2010;17:35–41.
10. Hakenewerth AM, Tintinalli JE, Waller AE, et al. Emergency department visits by patients with mental health disorders–North Carolina, 2008-2010. Available at: www.cdc.gov/mmwr/preview/mmwrhtml/mm6223a4.htm.
11. Wilson MP, Zeller SL. Introduction: reconsidering psychiatry in the emergency department. J Emerg Med 2012;43:771–2.
12. Dennis M, Beach M, Evans PA, et al. An examination of the accident and emergency management of deliberate self harm. J Accid Emerg Med 1997;14(5): 311–5.
13. Zun LS. Pitfalls in the care of the psychiatric patient in the emergency department. J Emerg Med 2012;43:829–35.
14. Baraff LJ, Janowicz N, Asarnow JR. Survey of California emergency departments about practices for management of suicidal patients and resources available for their care. Ann Emerg Med 2006;48:452–8.
15. Dolan MA, The Committee on Pediatric Emergency Medicine. Technical report–pediatric and adolescent mental health emergencies in the emergency medical services system. Pediatrics 2011;127:E1356–66.
16. Sills MR, Bland SD. Summary statistics for pediatric visits to US emergency departments, 1993-1999. Pediatrics 2002;110:E40.
17. Zun LS. Evidence-based evaluation of psychiatric patients. J Emerg Med 2005; 28:25–39.
18. Reeves RR, Perry CL, Burke RS. What does "medical clearance" for psychiatry really mean? J Psychosoc Nurs Ment Health Serv 2010;48:2–4.
19. Tintinalli JE, Peacock FW, Wright MA. Emergency medical evaluation of psychiatric patients. Ann Emerg Med 1994;23:859–62.
20. Weissberg MP. Emergency room medical clearance: an educational problem. Am J Psychiatry 1979;136:787–90.
21. Druss BG, von Esenwein SA, Compton MT, et al. Budget impact and sustainability of medical care management for persons with serious mental illness. Am J Psychiatry 2011;168:1171–8.
22. Kisely S, Sadek J, MacKenzie A, et al. Excess cancer mortality in psychiatric patients. Can J Psychiatry 2008;53:753–61.
23. Kisely S, Preston N, Xiao J, et al. Reducing all-cause mortality among patients with psychiatric disorders: a population-based study. CMAJ 2013;185: E50–6.
24. Dickerson FB, Stallings C, Origoni A, et al. Predictors of occupational status six months after hospitalization in persons with a recent onset of psychosis. Psychiatry Res 2008;160:278–84.

25. American Psychiatric Association Steering Committee on Practice Guidelines. Psychiatric evaluation of adults, a quick reference guide. Arlington (VA): American Psychiatric Association Practice Guidelines; 2006. p. 1–18.

26. American Psychiatric Association. American Psychiatric Association practice guidelines for the treatment of psychiatric disorders: compendium 2006. Arlington (VA): American Psychiatric Publication; 2006.

27. Lukens TW, Wolf SJ, Edlow JA, et al. Clinical policy: critical issues in the diagnosis and management of the adult psychiatric patient in the emergency department. Ann Emerg Med 2006;47:79–99.

28. Williams ER, Shepherd SM. Medical clearance of psychiatric patients. Emerg Med Clin North Am 2000;18:185–98.

29. Baren JM, Mace SE, Hendry PL, et al. Children's mental health emergencies-part 2: emergency department evaluation and treatment of children with mental health disorders. Pediatr Emerg Care 2008;24:485–98.

30. Bauer J, Roberts MR, Reisdorff EJ. Evaluation of behavioral and cognitive changes: the mental status examination. Emerg Med Clin North Am 1991; 9:1–12.

31. Hall RC, Popkin MK, Devaul RA, et al. Physical illness presenting as psychiatric disease. Arch Gen Psychiatry 1978;35:1315–20.

32. Biancosino B, Vanni A, Marmai L, et al. Factors related to admission of psychiatric patients to medical wards from the general hospital emergency department: a 3-year study of urgent psychiatric consultations. Int J Psychiatry Med 2009;39: 133–46.

33. Carlson RJ, Nayar N, Suh M. Psychiatric disorders among emergency psychiatric patients. Can J Psychiatry 1981;26:65–7.

34. Karas S. Behavioral emergencies: differentiating medical from psychiatric disease. Emerg Med Pract 2002;4:1–18.

35. Macalpine I, Hunter R. The "insanity" of King George III: a classic case of porphyria. Br Med J 1966;1.

36. Evans DL. Bipolar disorder: diagnostic challenges and treatment considerations. J Clin Psychiatry 2000;61:26–31.

37. Frame DS, Kercher EE. Acute psychosis. Functional versus organic. Emerg Med Clin North Am 1991;9:123–36.

38. Larson EW, Richelson E. Organic causes of mania. Mayo Clinic Proc 1988;63: 906–12.

39. Henneman PL, Mendoza R, Lewis RJ. Prospective evaluation of the emergency department medical clearance. Ann Emerg Med 1994;24:672–7.

40. Kakuma R, du Fort GG, Arsenault L, et al. Delirium in older emergency department patients discharged home: effect on survival. J Am Geriatr Soc 2003;51: 443–50.

41. Irons MJ, Farace E, Brady WJ, et al. Mental status screening of emergency department patients: normative study of the quick confusion scale. Acad Emerg Med 2002;9:989–94.

42. Sokal J, Messias E, Dickerson FB, et al. Comorbidity of medical illness among adults with serious mental illness who are receiving community psychiatric services. The J Nervous Ment Dis 2004;192:421–7.

43. Koita J, Riggio S, Jagoda A. The mental status examination in emergency practice. Emerg Med Clin North Am 2010;28:439–51.

44. Gregory RJ, Nihalani ND, Rodriguez E. Medical screening in the emergency department for psychiatric admissions: a procedural analysis. Gen Hosp Psychiatry 2004;26:405–10.

45. Szpakowicz M, Herd A. "Medically cleared": how well are patients with psychiatric presentations examined by emergency physicians? J Emerg Med 2008;35: 369–72.
46. Reeves RR, Pendarvis EJ, Kimble R. Unrecognized medical emergencies admitted to psychiatric units. Am J Emerg Med 2000;4:390–3.
47. Riba M, Hale M. Medical clearance: fact or fiction in the hospital emergency room. Psychosomatics 1990;30:400–4.
48. Reeves RR, Parker JD, Burke RS. Unrecognized physical illness prompting psychiatric admission. Ann Clin Psychiatry 2010;22:180–5.
49. Shah SJ, Fiorito M, McNamara RM. A screening tool to medically clear psychiatric patients in the emergency department. J Emerg Med 2012;43:871–5.
50. Hoffman RS. Diagnostic errors in the evaluation of behavioral disorders. JAMA 1982;248:964–7.
51. Korn CS, Currier GW, Henderson SO. "Medical clearance" of psychiatric patients without medical complaints in the emergency department. J Emerg Med 2000;18: 173–6.
52. Olshaker JS, Browne B, Jerrard DA. Medical clearance and screening of psychiatric patients in the emergency department. Acad Emerg Med 1997;4:124–8.
53. Donofrio JJ, Santillanes G, McCammack BD, et al. Clinical utility of screening laboratory tests in pediatric psychiatric patents presenting to the emergency department for medical clearance. Ann Emerg Med 2014;63(6):666–75.
54. Feldman L, Chen Y. The utility and financial implications of obtaining routing laboratory screening upon admission for child and adolescent psychiatric inpatients. J Psychiatr Pract 2011;17:375–81.
55. Santillanes G, Donofrio JJ, Lam CN, et al. Is medical clearance necessary for pediatric psychiatric patients? J Emerg Med 2014;46:800–7.
56. Sheline Y, Kehr C. Cost and utility of routine admission laboratory testing for psychiatric patients. Gen Hosp Psychiatry 1990;12:329–34.

Stabilization and Management of the Acutely Agitated or Psychotic Patient

Nathan Deal, MD[a], Michelle Hong, MD, PharmD[a],*,
Anu Matorin, MD[b], Asim A. Shah, MD[c]

KEYWORDS

- Agitation • Psychomotor agitation • Psychosis • Benzodiazepines • Antipsychotics

KEY POINTS

- Management strategies should use the least restrictive interventions for the shortest duration possible.
- The use of pharmacologic agents is not to simply render a patient unconscious, but rather to control agitation and aggression to circumvent violence and facilitate further assessment of the patient.
- Lorazepam is the preferred agent for the treatment of undifferentiated acute agitation.
- Seclusion and mechanical restraints are coercive measures that should be considered methods of last resort.

INTRODUCTION

As any emergency personnel can attest, the acutely agitated or psychotic patient is no stranger to the emergency department (ED). Often they present with little or no history, but clinicians and staff are nevertheless challenged to make decisions regarding how to best manage these patients. In addition to being agitated, an acutely psychotic patient may present with hallucinations or delusions that can further

Disclosures: None.
[a] Section of Emergency Medicine, Emergency Center, Ben Taub General Hospital, Baylor College of Medicine, 1504 Taub Loop, Room EC 61, Houston, TX 77030, USA; [b] Department of Psychiatry and Behavioral Sciences, Neuropsychiatric Center, Ben Taub General Hospital, Baylor College of Medicine, 1502 Taub Loop, Room 2.126, Houston, TX 77030, USA; [c] Department of Psychiatry and Behavioral Sciences, Neuropsychiatric Center, Ben Taub General Hospital, Baylor College of Medicine, 1502 Taub Loop, Room 2.125, Houston, TX 77030, USA
* Corresponding author.
E-mail address: Michelle.Chan@bcm.edu

Emerg Med Clin N Am 33 (2015) 739–752
http://dx.doi.org/10.1016/j.emc.2015.07.003
0733-8627/15/$ – see front matter © 2015 Elsevier Inc. All rights reserved.

emed.theclinics.com

complicate patient care because of poor insight and lack of cooperation.[1] When left untreated, an acutely agitated or psychotic patient can rapidly progress to hostile and violent behavior.

According to the US Bureau of Labor Statistics, there is an increasing trend of violent acts toward workers in the health care and social assistance industries, with nonfatal incidences occurring almost 5 times more often than in all other industries combined.[2] There is also evidence to suggest that many instances of assault go unreported.[3–5] Within the hospital itself, EDs are among the most common settings for violence to occur,[6] with some studies showing that more than 70% of emergency staff report being the victim of at least 1 violent act over a 1-year period.[7,8]

Psychosis is a syndrome that impairs a patient's ability to interact appropriately with reality. According to the *Diagnostic and Statistical Manual of Mental Disorders*, 5th edition (DSM-5), a defining feature of psychotic disorders is abnormal motor behavior, which can involve unpredictable agitation. DSM-5 goes on to define psychomotor agitation as excessive motor activity associated with a feeling of inner tension.[9] Cohen-Mansfield and Billig[10] defined agitation as "inappropriate verbal, vocal, or motor activity that is, not judged by an outside observer to result directly from the needs or confusion of the agitated individual." Regardless of the definition, the key concept to understand is that agitation is a symptom[10,11] of many medical and psychiatric disorders that can manifest itself both verbally and physically along a spectrum of severity. As a result, not all presentations of agitation require emergency intervention. To help determine which presentations warrant intervention, an expert consensus described 5 features that define clinically significant agitation.[12]

1. Abnormal and excessive verbal behavior such as shouting, cursing, threatening, or screaming
2. Abnormal and excessive physically aggressive behavior such as pushing, shoving, actively resisting care, repeatedly attempting to elope, or excessive threatening gestures
3. Heightened arousal
4. Symptoms cause clinically significant disruption of patient's functioning
5. Abnormal excessive or purposeless motor behavior

Ultimately these are all behaviors that are dynamic in nature, with several studies supporting the predictive value of agitation for subsequent aggressive or violent behavior,[13] in contrast to the traditional approach of assessing static risk factors for violent behavior such as history of prior violence, substance abuse, and certain psychiatric disorders including schizophrenia, borderline or antisocial personality disorder, acute mania, and psychotic depression,[14] information which may not be immediately available in the emergency setting.

PATHOPHYSIOLOGY

Although the pathophysiology of agitation is not well elucidated, it is thought to be due to the imbalance of certain neurotransmitters, particularly serotonin, dopamine, norepinephrine, and γ-aminobutyric acid (GABA).[15,16] In particular, increases in serotonin or GABA, or decreases in dopamine or norepinephrine, can lead to or contribute to agitation.[15] The variability in presentation is in part due to the many organic and inorganic causes of agitation. Well-established causes of agitation are listed in **Box 1**. In addition, many other unusual but potential causes of acute agitation or psychosis in the ED have been reported in the literature, including

---

Box 1
Causes of agitation

Neurologic

  Brain tumors (limbic, hypothalamic)

  Cerebral vascular accident

  Dementia (Alzheimer, Huntington, Parkinson)

  Intracranial hemorrhage

  Traumatic brain injury

Cardiopulmonary: hypoxia

Infectious: encephalitis, meningitis, sepsis

Metabolic

  Endocrine: diabetic ketoacidosis, hypoglycemia, temperature dysregulation, thyroid dysfunction

  Electrolyte imbalance: hypercalcemia, hypernatremia, hyponatremia

  Vitamin deficiencies: niacin, thiamine

Substance related

  Alcohol

  Hallucinogens (phencyclidine)

  Steroids

  Stimulants (amphetamines, bath salts, cocaine)

  Synthetic marijuana

Psychiatric

  Antisocial personality disorder

  Brief psychotic disorder

  Bipolar disorder

  Borderline personality disorder

  Posttraumatic stress disorder

  Psychotic depression

  Schizophrenia

---

cardiac myxoma,[17] diphenhydramine,[18,19] γ-hydroxybutyrate,[20] and synthetic cannabinoids.[21]

ASSESSMENT

Emergency personnel tend to enjoy and thrive in the controlled chaos of the ED. However, to patients and their families, the chaotic nature of the ED is not as enjoyable and may appear much less controlled as patients get shuffled from one location to the next, each place a flurry of activity. The noise, activity, crowding, and potentially long waits create the perfect medium for agitation and psychosis to manifest.[22] So although patients may present acutely agitated, it is important to recognize that some patients may develop agitation while in the ED. Moreover, although the patient who becomes acutely agitated during the ED visit may have more background and medical history available compared with the patient who is agitated on arrival, the initial assessment of both patients remains the same.

When called to the bedside of an acutely agitated patient, physicians should immediately and inherently perform a risk assessment for violence to ensure the safety of both the patient and staff. Although studies suggest that clinicians are not good predictors of patient violence,[23–25] physicians should never minimize clinical gestalt.[26,27] Aside from assessing the presence and severity of previously mentioned dynamic factors, the presence of static factors may heighten the perceived risk of violence. Although it may not be immediately possible or practical to ask patients about a history of violence, homicidal or suicidal ideation/intent, or substance abuse, it is important to directly address these issues at some point during the initial assessment.[26,28]

Once safety is established, the next step, as with any patient, is to conduct a primary survey, including the review of vital signs and full exposure of the patient. Not only does this aid in the visual assessment for overt signs of injury but also offers the opportunity to check for concealed weapons.[28,29] Other important parts of the initial evaluation include a quick but thorough neurologic examination and a finger-stick to assess for hypoglycemia. Although understanding the cause of agitation may aid in the long-term management of an acutely agitated patient, the purpose of the initial assessment is not to obtain a diagnosis but rather to diffuse potentially violent situations and treat serious or life-threatening conditions.[22]

Collateral information from family or emergency medical services personnel pertaining to the events leading up to the patient's presentation is always of value. However, although a thorough history is important, one must be wary of bias, particularly toward psychiatric causes of acute agitation and psychosis in patients with known psychiatric histories. Many documented cases in the literature indicate how acute agitation or psychosis may be prematurely misdiagnosed as primarily psychiatric when the underlying etiology is organic.[30–33]

Several signs and symptoms may help distinguish organic and potentially life-threatening causes of agitation or psychosis from inorganic causes. Increased suspicion for an underlying medical condition warranting additional investigation should be considered in the presence of any of the items noted in **Box 2**.[28,34,35]

Often it is not possible to conduct an initial history and physical because of the patient's presenting condition, in which case one is faced with managing a patient with acute undifferentiated agitation.

Box 2
Signs and symptoms associated with organic causes of agitation and psychosis

Abnormal vital signs

Focal neurologic deficits

Signs of trauma

Disorientation

Impaired cognition

Nonauditory hallucinations

Impaired speech

Fluctuating symptoms

MANAGEMENT GOALS

The short-term goals of managing an acutely agitated or psychotic patient are early recognition, stabilization of life-threatening conditions, and rapid control of agitation or psychosis, ideally by calming the patient without undue force or inducing significant sedation to prevent or minimize harm to the patient or others.[1,12,13,36] Ultimately the goal of emergency care is to exclude organic causes of agitation or psychosis, and foster appropriate and timely disposition. Calming the patient without oversedation facilitates further assessment, especially for the patient in whom prior assessment could not be completed because of agitation or psychosis. Although oversedation will result in a calmer patient, it is not without its side effects and may delay the ability for further assessment, potentially prolonging the length of stay in the ED.[16,37]

These short-term goals can be accomplished by several different methods or a combination of methods, depending on the acuity and severity of the situation. Management tactics can be divided into pharmacologic and nonpharmacologic. Nonpharmacologic strategies include environmental interventions, de-escalation techniques, and mechanical restraints. In general, the management of acutely agitated or psychotic patients should begin with the least restrictive measure before proceeding to more restrictive measures. Mechanical restraints are considered the most restrictive method of management, and should only be used for patients in whom all other methods have proved ineffective in maintaining the safety of the patient or others.[12,26,38,39] Whenever possible, physicians should elicit patient input and attempt to make patients active participants in their own care, rather than use coercive measures.

NONPHARMACOLOGIC STRATEGIES
Environmental Intervention

Creating an environment that promotes safety and minimizes stimulation of an agitated or psychotic patient can be particularly difficult in the ED, where personnel are always on the move and environments may change as patients are shuffled from the waiting room to triage to a bed. Despite these challenges, a few fundamental strategies should be applied regardless of the situation. Aside from screening patients for weapons, it is important to also remove any objects with the potential to become a weapon, including pens, chairs, and personal effects.[26,40] Maintaining adequate staffing and training staff to recognize and manage agitated or violent patients is also a key component in promoting safety.[36,41] Although some EDs offer individual rooms that can minimize environmental stimuli from noise and activity, every ED should maintain an area that offers a quiet, less stimulating space for patients when necessary.[26,28,36]

Seclusion and Mechanical Restraints

Seclusion and mechanical restraints are considered coercive measures,[11,13,38] with seclusion typically defined as involuntary confinement.[42,43] The utility of seclusion in the management of acutely agitated patients is questionable,[42,44] but remains a common intervention.[45,46] In addition, seclusion and mechanical restraints are not without their risks, and have been associated with both physical and psychological adverse effects.[28,42,44]

Both mechanical restraints and seclusion should be considered methods of last resort. Between the 2 options, seclusion is considered the less restrictive choice. As with any coercive measure, seclusion and mechanical restraints should never be used as a convenience for emergency personnel or as punishment to the patient. Ultimately it may be best to think of seclusion and mechanical restraints as the result of treatment failures rather than as therapeutic options.[47]

De-Escalation Techniques

In conjunction with providing a safe and calm environment, de-escalation techniques are considered first-line strategies in the management of acutely agitated or psychotic patients who are not imminently in danger of hurting themselves or others. In addition to nonviolent behavior, de-escalation techniques work best in the agitated, but cooperative patient.

De-escalation involves both verbal and nonverbal strategies to help calm a patient. The first step in successfully de-escalating a patient is to establish rapport. Recognizing and addressing basic needs is a simple but effective way to accomplish this. Reassuring that the patient is in a safe environment, offering food and water, and providing blankets addresses safety, hunger, and comfort.[13,14,40,45,48] Often overlooked, but equally important is ensuring adequate pain control.[28]

According to the American Psychiatric Association Task Force on Psychiatric Emergency Services, staff should receive annual training in managing behavioral emergencies in the least restrictive manner, and continuous training in alternatives to seclusion and restraints.[36] In a survey of EDs in the United States, 76% of emergency personnel reported some training on alternatives to pharmacologic and mechanical restraints.[45] In a separate survey, approximately 80% of emergency nurses attended ED violence prevention/diffusion training, with 50% of hospitals requiring some form of training.[49] Although a literature search revealed no published clinical trials regarding effective de-escalation techniques in the emergency setting, the literature does describe some common strategies.[13,40,50] These approaches include maintaining a calm and respectful demeanor, being mindful of personal space, avoiding threatening or confrontational behavior (avoid crossing arms, standing over patient, or prolonged eye contact), and showing empathy. Important verbal techniques include addressing violence directly, setting limits, offering choices, and informing the patient of the consequences of poor or inappropriate behavior.

PHARMACOLOGIC STRATEGIES

When environmental intervention and de-escalation efforts fail, the next step in management is the use of pharmacologic agents. An ideal agent would be fast acting, cost effective, well tolerated, noninvasive, and sedating, with minimal drug interactions.[12,13,51,52] These agents can be used as monotherapy or in combination, and can be administered in a variety of formulations including oral liquids, tablets, rapidly disintegrating tablets, intravenous and intramuscular medications, and newer inhalational agents.[53,54] In cooperative patients oral medications are preferred, as they are less invasive and traumatic. For less cooperative and more agitated patients, parenteral agents are often used.

Rapid tranquilization refers to the use of parenteral medications (**Table 1**) in a stepwise approach for the management of acute behavioral emergencies.[11,55] This term was used by Dubin in the 1980s to describe the interval dosing of antipsychotics and benzodiazepines to quickly calm the severely agitated or hostile patient.[55,56] Despite the frequent use of antipsychotics for this purpose, rapid tranquilization may be used in patients without a psychiatric diagnosis, and is not intended to be a treatment for underlying psychosis. Although benzodiazepines are sedating agents, the goal of rapid tranquilization should not be to render a patient unconscious, but rather to control agitation and aggression to circumvent violence and facilitate further assessment of the patient.

Though typically reserved for the chronic management of agitation and aggression, the use of other agents such as β-blockers, mood stabilizers, and selective serotonin reuptake inhibitors in the setting of acute agitation has been described.

Table 1			
Parenteral options for acute agitation			
	Onset (min)[a]	Initial Dose[b] (mg)	Considerations
Benzodiazepines			
Diazepam	30	5–10 IV	Avoid IM because of unpredictable absorption. Useful in the setting of alcohol withdrawal
Lorazepam	2–5 IV 15–30 IM	1–2 IM/IV	—
Midazolam	120 IV 4–6 h IM	2.5–5	Higher risk of respiratory depression compared with lorazepam and diazepam
Antipsychotics			
Aripiprazole	60	9.75	Relatively safe side-effect profile
Haloperidol	1–2 IV 30–60 IM	5 IM/IV	Risk for EPS. Higher risk of QT prolongation, particularly if given IV. IV haloperidol is an off-label route and requires careful monitoring for cardiac arrhythmias if used
Olanzapine	15–45	10	Use with caution when given with BDZ because of increased risk of cardiopulmonary depression
Ziprasidone	30–45	20	Low risk of QT prolongation

Abbreviations: BDZ, benzodiazepine; EPS, extrapyramidal symptoms; IM, intramuscular; IV, intravenous.
[a] Values listed as minutes unless otherwise specified.
[b] IM doses listed unless otherwise specified.

Benzodiazepines

Benzodiazepines are a group of sedative-hypnotic agents that act on $GABA_A$ receptors in the central nervous system. In addition to sedation and hypnosis, they also have anxiolytic, anticonvulsant, and amnestic properties. Benzodiazepines are typically categorized according to their elimination half-lives into short-, intermediate-, and long-acting agents. Lorazepam, an intermediate-acting benzodiazepine, is the most frequently used drug of its class for the management of acute agitation.[12,13] Lorazepam is a particularly useful agent for the treatment of undifferentiated agitation or psychosis in the ED because of its wide availability, relatively rapid onset, ease of administration, and multifaceted pharmacologic effects. In addition, lorazepam may be used to treat anxiety or alcohol withdrawal, both of which can co-occur or contribute to agitation.

Although it is not approved by the US Food and Drug Administration (FDA) for acute agitation, lorazepam is typically administered intramuscularly or orally, with studies suggesting that it is effective at single doses ranging from 0.5 to 3 mg.[12,57,58] Although the evidence is modest, lorazepam seems to be at least as effective as haloperidol with reportedly fewer side effects.[57,58] It can also be given in combination with haloperidol.[59,60] In fact, studies consistently show that a combination of a benzodiazepine plus an antipsychotic is more effective than when either agent is used alone.[61,62]

Midazolam is a short-acting benzodiazepine that is gaining popularity because of its faster onset and shorter duration of sedation in comparison with lorazepam.[63] However, it should be used cautiously in acutely agitated patients who appear cirrhotic or present with alcohol intoxication. Although both lorazepam and midazolam are metabolized by the liver, lorazepam predominantly undergoes glucuronidation, which is a less affected process in mild to moderate cirrhosis.[64] By contrast, the use of mid-azolam in patients with cirrhosis is associated with a significant increase in duration of action.

Antipsychotics

Antipsychotics are commonly divided into 2 categories based on their mechanism of action and clinical profile. First-generation antipsychotics include the butyrophenones haloperidol and droperidol. Also known as typical antipsychotics, these agents block dopamine receptors in the brain, and as a class are associated with extrapyramidal side effects. Second-generation, or atypical, antipsychotics antagonize both seroto-nin and dopamine receptors, but affect dopamine to a lesser degree than their prede-cessors, resulting in fewer extrapyramidal effects.[65] Of the atypical antipsychotics, oral risperidone or olanzapine and intramuscular ziprasidone or olanzapine are commonly selected as the initial choice in managing acute agitation or psychosis.[12]

Collectively, physicians have the most experience with haloperidol regarding the use of antipsychotics for patients with acute agitation or psychosis in the emergency setting. As previously mentioned, haloperidol is commonly used in combination with a benzodiazepine such as lorazepam. However, there is a strong drive toward more frequent use of atypical antipsychotics as the result of a perceived improvement in their side-effect profiles.

Droperidol is an alternative that has been studied as a single agent in comparison with benzodiazepines. In a prospective randomized trial versus lorazepam, droperidol was shown to have faster onset and more consistent sedation with less likelihood of repeat dosing.[66] In a more recent randomized controlled trial, droperidol was compared with midazolam. Each drug was given 5 mg intravenously every 5 minutes until sedation was achieved. The investigators found no difference between the drugs in terms of onset and efficacy, but midazolam was associated with an increased risk for airway complications.[67] In a third, similarly sized study, droperidol was compared with ziprasidone and midazolam. The investigators concluded that droperidol and ziprasidone were superior to midazolam in terms of adequate sedation; however, they did note that onset of action was slower with droperidol than with either of the other 2 agents.[68] A 2001 black-box warning issued against droperidol because of con-cerns for significant risk of cardiac arrhythmias and, more recently, lack of availability resulting from manufacturer-suspended distribution now limits its role.

Novel Agents

Ketamine is an N-methyl-D-aspartate receptor antagonist with amnestic properties, traditionally categorized as a general anesthetic agent. Although it has a history dating back to the 1960s, in the past decade ketamine has garnered increasing interest as a rapid tranquilizer in the prehospital setting. Several case series[69–71] ranging from 2 to 18 patients involving the use of ketamine in the prehospital setting, and 1 case report from the ED[72] seem to suggest that ketamine is both effective and safe, with no wors-ening of agitation. However, in a case series of 13 patients who received prehospital ketamine for chemical restraint, 10 of 12 patients presented to the ED in moderate to deep sedation. In this small group, ketamine use was associated with hypoxia, laryng-ospasm, and emergence reactions.[73] As ketamine is also used for rapid sequence intubation, it is prudent to mentally prepare for the potential need for respiratory sup-port. Although it seems counterintuitive for a drug well known for its psychotropic ef-fects to be used for agitation, mechanistically the rapid onset of action of ketamine and its indirect effects on dopamine release may prove useful.[65] It is unlikely that ketamine will become a routine agent in the management of acute agitation or psychosis, given that it does not meet the ideal criteria of being nonsedating. However, its use in the rapid take-down of patients who are at imminent danger to themselves or others is yet to be determined, as studies thus far are too small to support its routine use.

Loxapine is another older agent gaining new life in the form of an inhaled powder.[74] Loxapine is considered a first-generation antipsychotic but, like second-generation agents, it also has some activity against serotonin receptors. The inhaled formulation is currently approved by the FDA for the acute treatment of agitation associated with schizophrenia or bipolar I disorder. Unfortunately, the use of inhaled loxapine requires patient cooperation and coordination for proper administration, potentially limiting its usefulness in the acute and emergent setting.

Other possible pharmacologic strategies to consider are the use of intranasally administered agents. Studies suggest that the use of intranasal haloperidol or lorazepam results in higher peak levels and faster absorption rates in comparison with intramuscular administration.[75,76]

SUMMARY

Much of current clinical practice in the management of acutely agitated or psychotic patients is based on anecdotal evidence and expert opinion. At present, the general

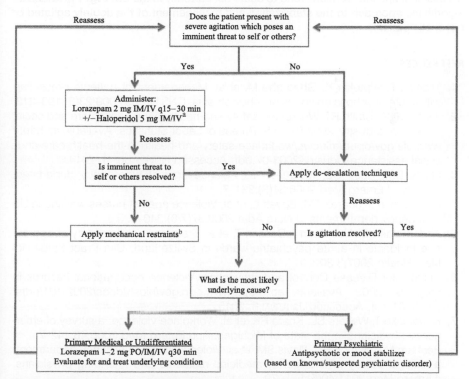

Fig. 1. Approach to acute agitation. [a]The routine use of anticholinergic agents may result in oversedation. Anticholinergics such as diphenhydramine and benztropine should be limited to use in the setting of extrapyramidal symptoms. [b]Requires frequent reassessment and appropriate documentation with the goal of maintaining the least restrictive restraints for the least amount of time. IM, intramuscular; IV, intravenous; PO, by mouth; q, every.

approach to managing the acutely agitated or psychotic patient consists of creating and maintaining a safe and calming environment to the furthest extent possible, in addition to the use of various de-escalation techniques. In patients who continue to remain agitated despite these strategies, pharmacologic agents should be initiated to prevent acutely agitated patients from harming themselves or others.

Unfortunately, many studies aimed at the pharmacologic management of acute agitation have been small and lack the power needed to show advantages in use. In fact, although benzodiazepines are commonly used as single agents,[12] a Cochrane Review evaluating the efficacy of benzodiazepines alone or in combination with other agents for psychosis-induced aggression or agitation failed to find sufficient evidence to support or refute this practice.[77] Nonetheless, current guidelines suggest that benzodiazepines can be considered for monotherapy in mild to moderate agitation or agitation related to alcohol withdrawal for those patients in whom underlying psychosis is not suspected.[12]

Antipsychotics may also be used as monotherapy for mild to moderate agitation, and should be considered particularly in patients with active psychosis or known psychiatric history. Combination therapy and rapid tranquilization should be considered for patients who present with moderate to severe agitation. Coercive techniques such as seclusion and mechanical restraints are methods of last resort, and should only be considered when all other treatment options have been exhausted. Although assessment and interventions tend to occur concurrently in the ED, **Fig. 1** provides an algorithmic approach to the stabilization and management of the acutely agitated or psychotic patient.

REFERENCES

1. Thomas P, Alptekin K, Gheorghe M, et al. Management of patients presenting with acute psychotic episodes of schizophrenia. CNS Drugs 2009;23(3):193–212.
2. Janocha JA, Smith RT. Workplace safety and health in the health care and social assistance industry, 2003-07. U.S. Bureau of Labor Statistics. Available at: http://www.bls.gov/opub/mlr/cwc/workplace-safety-and-health-in-the-health-care-and-social-assistance-industry-2003-07.pdf. Accessed November 3, 2014.
3. Gates DM, Ross CS, McQueen L. Violence against emergency department workers. J Emerg Med 2006;31(3):331–7.
4. Gacki-Smith J, Juarez AM, Boyett L, et al. Violence against nurses working in US emergency departments. J Nurs Adm 2009;37(7/8):340–9.
5. Abderhalden C, Needham I, Dassen T, et al. Frequency and severity of aggressive incidents in acute psychiatric wards in Switzerland. Clin Pract Epidemiol Ment Health 2007;3:30.
6. Centers for Disease Control and Prevention. Violence occupational hazards in hospitals. 2002. Available at: http://www.cdc.gov/niosh/docs/2002-101/pdfs/2002-101.pdf. Accessed January 6, 2015.
7. Kowalenko T, Walters BL, Khare RK, et al. Workplace violence: a survey of emergency physicians in the state of Michigan. Ann Emerg Med 2005;46:142–7.
8. Benham M, Tillotson RD, Davis SM, et al. Violence in the emergency department: a national survey of emergency medicine residents and attending physicians. J Emerg Med 2011;40(5):565–79.
9. American Psychiatric Association. Diagnostic and statistical manual of mental disorders. 5th edition. Washington, DC: 2013.
10. Cohen-Mansfield J, Billig N. Agitated behaviors in the elderly. I. A conceptual review. J Am Geriatr Soc 1986;34(10):711–21.

11. Rocca P, Villari V, Bogetto F. Managing the aggressive and violent patient in the psychiatric emergency. Prog Neuropsychopharmacol Biol Psychiatry 2006;30:586–98.
12. Allen MH, Currier GW, Carpenter D, et al. The expert consensus panel for behavioral emergencies 2005. J Psychiatr Pract 2005;11(Suppl 1):4–112.
13. Hankin CS, Bronstone A, Koran LM. Agitation in the inpatient psychiatric setting: a review of clinical presentation, burden, and treatment. J Psychiatr Pract 2011; 17(3):170–85.
14. Coburn VA, Mycyk MB. Physical and chemical restraints. Emerg Med Clin North Am 2009;27(4):655–67.
15. Lindenmayer JP. The pathophysiology of agitation. J Clin Psychiatry 2000; 61(Suppl 14):5–10.
16. Citrome L. New treatments for agitation. Psychiatr Q 2004;75(3):197–213.
17. Jain RS, Nagpal K, Jain R, et al. Acute psychosis presenting as a sole manifestation of left atrial myxoma: a new paradigm. Am J Emerg Med 2014;32(12):1556.
18. Christensen RC. Misdiagnosis of anticholinergic delirium as schizophrenic psychosis. Am J Emerg Med 1995;13(1):117–8.
19. Sexton JD, Pronchik DJ. Diphenhydramine-induced psychosis with therapeutic doses. Am J Emerg Med 1997;15(5):548–9.
20. Zvosec DL, Smith SW. Agitation is common in γ-hydroxybutyrate toxicity. Am J Emerg Med 2005;23:316–20.
21. Rodgman CR, Kinzie E, Leimbach E. Bad mojo: use of the new marijuana substitute leads to more and more ED visits for acute psychosis. Am J Emerg Med 2011;29(2):232.
22. Citrome L, Volavka J. Violent patients in the emergency setting. Psychiatr Clin North Am 1999;22(4):789–801.
23. Lidz CW, Mulvey EP, Gardner W. The accuracy of predictions of violence to others. JAMA 1993;269(8):1007–11.
24. Haim R, Rabinowitz J, Lereya J, et al. Predictions made by psychiatrists and psychiatric nurses of violence by patients. Psychiatr Serv 2002;53(5):622–4.
25. Serper MR, Goldberg BR, Herman KG, et al. Predictors of aggression on the psychiatric inpatient service. Compr Psychiatry 2005;46(2):121–7.
26. Petit JR. Management of the acutely violent patient. Psychiatr Clin North Am 2005;28:701–11.
27. Rice MM, Moore GP. Management of the violent patient. Therapeutic and legal considerations. Emerg Med Clin North Am 1991;9(1):13–30.
28. Rossi J, Swan MC, Isaacs ED. The violent or agitated patient. Emerg Med Clin North Am 2010;28:235–56.
29. Karas S. Behavior emergencies: differentiating medical from psychiatric disease. Emerg Med Pract 2002;4(3):1–20.
30. Tintinalli JE, Peacock FW, Wright MA. Emergency medical evaluation of psychiatric patients. Ann Emerg Med 1994;23(4):859–62.
31. Duwe BV, Turetsky BI. Misdiagnosis of schizophrenia in a patient with psychotic symptoms. Neuropsychiatry Neuropsychol Behav Neurol 2002;15(4):252–60.
32. Brda D, Tang EC. Visual hallucinations from retinal detachment misdiagnosed as psychosis. J Psychiatr Pract 2011;17(2):133–6.
33. Nia S. Psychiatric signs and symptoms in treatable inborn errors of metabolism. J Neurol 2014;261(Suppl 2):S559–68.
34. Sood TR, Mcstay CM. Evaluation of the psychiatric patient. Emerg Med Clin North Am 2009;27(4):669–83.
35. Nordstrom K, Zun LS, Wilson MP, et al. Medical evaluation and triage of the agitated patient: consensus statement of the American Association for

Emergency Psychiatry Project BETA Medical Evaluation Workgroup. West J Emerg Med 2012;13:3–10.

36. Allen MH, Forster P, Zealberg J, et al. Report and recommendations regarding psychiatric emergency and crisis services. APA Task Force on Psychiatric Emergency Services 2002. Available at: http://www.emergencypsychiatry.org/data/tfr200201.pdf. Accessed January 6, 2015.

37. Wilson M, Pepper D, Currier G, et al. The psychopharmacology of agitation: consensus statement of the American Association for Emergency Psychiatry Project BETA Psychopharmacology Workgroup. West J Emerg Med 2012;13(1):26–34.

38. Annas GJ. The last resort—the use of physical restraints in medical emergencies. N Engl J Med 1999;341(18):1408–12.

39. Wise R. New restraint standards will change your practice. ED Manag 2000;12(8):93–5.

40. Richmond JS, Berlin JS, Fishkind AB, et al. Verbal de-escalation of the agitated patient: consensus statement of the American Association for Emergency Psychiatry Project BETA De-escalation Workgroup. West J Emerg Med 2012;13:17–25.

41. Occupational Safety & Health Administration. Guidelines for preventing workplace violence for health care & social service workers. Available at: https://www.osha.gov/Publications/OSHA3148/osha3148.html. Accessed November 19, 2014.

42. Huf G, Coutinho ESF, Adams CE. Physical restraints versus seclusion room for management of people with acute aggression or agitation due to psychotic illness (TREC-SAVE): a randomized trial. Psychol Med 2012;42:2265–73.

43. Knox DK, Holloman G. Use and avoidance of seclusion and restraint: consensus statement of the American Association for Emergency Psychiatry Project BETA Seclusion and Restraint Workgroup. West J Emerg Med 2012;13(1):35–40.

44. Nelstrop L, Chandler-Oatts J, Bingley W, et al. A systematic review of the safety and effectiveness of restraint and seclusion as interventions for the short-term management of violence in adult psychiatric inpatient settings and emergency departments. Worldviews Evid Based Nurs 2006;3(1):8–18.

45. Downey LVA, Zun LS, Gonzales SJ. Frequency of alternative to restraints and seclusion and uses of agitation reduction techniques in the emergency department. Gen Hosp Psychiatry 2007;29:470–4.

46. Zun LS, Downey L. The use of seclusion in emergency medicine. Gen Hosp Psychiatry 2005;27(5):365–71.

47. Smith GM, Davis RH, Bixler EO, et al. Pennsylvania state hospital system's seclusion and restraint reduction program. Psychiatr Serv 2005;56(9):1115–22.

48. Young GP. The agitated patient in the emergency department. Emerg Med Clin North Am 1987;5:765–81.

49. Emergency Nurses Association Institute for Emergency Nursing Research. Emergency department violence surveillance study. 2011. Available at: http://www.ena.org/practice-research/research/Documents/ENAEDVSReportNovember2011.pdf. Accessed December 7, 2014.

50. Hodge A, Andrea M. Violence and aggression in the emergency department: a critical care perspective. Aust Crit Care 2007;20(2):61–7.

51. Sorrentino A. Chemical restraints for the agitated, violent, or psychotic pediatric patient in the emergency department: controversies and recommendations. Curr Opin Pediatr 2004;16:201–5.

52. Zeller SL, Rhoades RW. Systematic reviews of assessment measures and pharmacologic treatments for agitation. Clin Ther 2010;32(3):403–25.

53. Nordstrom K, Allen MH. Alternative delivery systems for agents to treat acute agitation: progress to date. Drugs 2013;73:1783–92.

54. Loxapine inhalational powder (Adasuve) [package insert]. Horsham, PA: Teva Select Brands, a division of Teva Pharmaceuticals USA, Inc; 2013.

55. Chapter 10. Emergency department treatment. In: Schatzberg AF, Cole JO, DeBattista C, editors. Manual of clinical psychopharmacology. 7th edition. Arlington (VA): American Psychiatric Publishing, Inc; 2010.

56. Dubin WR, Feld JA. Rapid tranquilization of the violent patient. Am J Emerg Med 1989;7(3):313–20.

57. Salzman C, Solomon D, Miyawaki E, et al. Parenteral lorazepam versus parenteral haloperidol for the control of psychotic disruptive behavior. J Clin Psychiatry 1991;52:177–80.

58. Foster S, Kessel J, Berman ME, et al. Efficacy of lorazepam and haloperidol for rapid tranquilization in a psychiatric emergency room setting. Int Clin Psychopharmacol 1997;12:175–9.

59. Battaglia J, Moss S, Rush J, et al. Haloperidol, lorazepam, or both for psychotic agitation? A multicenter, prospective, double-blind, emergency department study. Am J Emerg Med 1997;15:335–40.

60. Garza-Trevino ES, Hollister LE, Overall JE, et al. Efficacy of combinations of intramuscular antipsychotics and sedative-hypnotics for control of psychotic agitation. Am J Psychiatry 1989;146:1598–601.

61. Chan EW, Taylor DM, Knott JC, et al. Intravenous droperidol or olanzapine as an adjunct to midazolam for the acutely agitated patient: a multicenter, randomized, double-blind, placebo-controlled clinical trial. Ann Emerg Med 2013;61(1): 72–81.

62. Bieniek SA, Ownby RL, Penalver A, et al. A double-blind study of lorazepam versus the combination of haloperidol and lorazepam in managing agitation. Pharmacotherapy 1998;18(1):57–62.

63. Nobay F, Simon BC, Levitt MA, et al. A prospective, double-blind, randomized trial of midazolam versus haloperidol versus lorazepam in the chemical restraint of violent and severely agitated patients. Acad Emerg Med 2004;11(7):744–9.

64. Verbeeck RK. Pharmacokinetics and dosage adjustment in patients with hepatic dysfunction. Eur J Clin Pharmacol 2008;64:1147–61.

65. Meyer JM. Chapter 16. Pharmacotherapy of psychosis and mania. In: Brunton LL, Chabner BA, Knollmann BC, editors. Goodman & Gilman's the pharmacological basis of therapeutics. 12th edition. New York: McGraw-Hill; 2011.

66. Richards JR, Derlet RW, Duncan DR. Chemical restraint for the agitated patient in the emergency department: lorazepam versus droperidol. J Emerg Med 1998; 16(4):567–73.

67. Knott JC, Taylor DM, Castle DJ. Randomized clinical trial comparing intravenous midazolam and droperidol for sedation of the acutely agitated patient in the emergency department. Ann Emerg Med 2006;47(1):61–7.

68. Martel M, Sterzinger A, Miner J, et al. Management of acute undifferentiated agitation in the emergency department: a randomized double-blind trial of droperidol, ziprasidone, and midazolam. Acad Emerg Med 2005;12(12): 1167–72.

69. Le Cong M, Gynther B, Hunter E, et al. Ketamine sedation for patients with acute agitation and psychiatric illness requiring aeromedical retrieval. Emerg Med J 2012;29(4):335–7.

70. Melamed E, Oron Y, Ben-Avraham R, et al. The combative multitrauma patient: a protocol for prehospital management. Eur J Emerg Med 2007;14(5):265–8.

71. Ho JD, Smith SW, Nystrom PC, et al. Successful management of excited delirium syndrome with prehospital ketamine: two case examples. Prehosp Emerg Care 2012;17:274–9.
72. Roberts JR, Geeting GK. Intramuscular ketamine for the rapid tranquilization of the uncontrollable, violent, and dangerous adult patient. J Trauma 2001;51: 1008–10.
73. Burnett AM, Salzman JG, Griffith KR, et al. The emergency department experience with prehospital ketamine: a case series of 13 patients. Prehosp Emerg Care 2012;16(4):553–9.
74. Keating GM. Loxapine inhalation powder: a review of its use in the acute treatment of agitation in patients with bipolar disorder or schizophrenia. CNS Drugs 2013;27(6):479–89.
75. Miller JL, Ashford JW, Archer SM, et al. Comparison of intranasal administration of haloperidol with intravenous and intramuscular administration: a pilot pharmacokinetic study. Pharmacotherapy 2008;28(7):875–82.
76. Wermeling DP, Miller JL, Archer SM, et al. Bioavailability and pharmacokinetics of lorazepam after intranasal, intravenous, and intramuscular administration. J Clin Pharmacol 2001;41(11):1225–31.
77. Gillies D, Smapson S, Beck A, et al. Benzodiazepines for psychosis-induced aggression or agitation. Cochrane Database Syst Rev 2013;(4):CD003079.

Stabilizing and Managing Patients with Altered Mental Status and Delirium

Ebelechukwu A. Odiari, MD[a],*, Navdeep Sekhon, MD[b],
Jin Y. Han, MD[c], Elizabeth H. David, MD[c]

KEYWORDS

- Altered mental status • Delirium • Emergency department • Management
- Antipsychotics

KEY POINTS

- Altered mental status is a common but nonspecific emergency department (ED) presentation that can signify underlying serious pathology.
- Delirium is a more defined mental status change caused by another medical condition, and carries a high morbidity and mortality if missed.
- The ED physician should maintain a high index of suspicion for delirium, because if missed in the ED, it is more likely to be missed on the wards as well.
- Management of delirium is directed toward treating the underlying course, with adjunctive use of antipsychotics and benzodiazepines for management of agitated delirium in the ED.

INTRODUCTION

Altered mental status (AMS) is a common, yet challenging, clinical presentation that emergency medicine physicians encounter. It is present in about 4% to 10% of ED patients[1] and can be seen in all patient populations, from pediatric to geriatric. It is a nonspecific term used to describe the whole spectrum of brain dysfunctions such as dementia, psychiatric disorder, and delirium. Clinical features of patients who are described as having AMS include: bizarre behavior, confusion, hyperalertness, obtundation, stupor, and frank coma. Of the brain dysfunctions that are largely described as

Disclosure Statement: The authors have nothing to disclose.
a Section of Emergency Medicine, Baylor College of Medicine, 1504 Taub Loop, Houston, TX 77030, USA; b Section of Emergency Medicine, Baylor College of Medicine, 439 Jackson Hill Street, Houston, TX 77007, USA; c Menninger Department of Psychiatry and Behavioral Sciences, Baylor College of Medicine, 1502 Taub Loop, NPC Building 2nd Floor, Houston, TX 77030, USA
* Corresponding author.
E-mail address: odiari@bcm.edu

Emerg Med Clin N Am 33 (2015) 753–764
http://dx.doi.org/10.1016/j.emc.2015.07.004
0733-8627/15/$ – see front matter Published by Elsevier Inc.

emed.theclinics.com

AMS, delirium carries the highest morbidity and mortality when missed.[2,3] However, emergency physicians miss delirium in 57% to 83% of the cases, because its clinical presentation can be subtle, there is time pressure, or perhaps because it is not sought.[4] Additionally, if the patient is admitted, more than 90% of delirium that is missed in the ED will also be missed in the hospital setting.[4,5] This article provides a practical approach to the recognition, stabilization, and management of AMS in the ED, with an emphasis on delirium.

RECOGNIZING DELIRIUM

Since delirium carries a high morbidity and mortality if missed, but can be subtle to recognize, several screening tools have been used in different clinical settings to facilitate this diagnosis. Some of the tools include Diagnostic and Statistical Manual of Mental Disorders, Fifth Edition (DSM-5) and confusion assessment method (CAM).

Based on the DSM-5 and CAM algorithm, delirium could be defined as an acute change in mental status from baseline with fluctuation in awareness, attention, and cognitive function, caused by a medical condition, substance intoxication, or withdrawal. These changes in cognitive function include perceptual disturbances, memory impairment, disorganized thinking, and disorientation. Delirium can also cause emotional symptoms, including anxiety and behavioral disturbance in addition to the changes in the sleep cycle. The DSM-5 criteria and the CAM algorithm for delirium are described in **Box 1** and **Fig 2**.

Box 1
Confusion assessment method algorithm

Feature 1: Acute Onset and Fluctuating Course

This feature is usually obtained from a family member or nurse and is shown by positive responses to the following questions:

Is there evidence of an acute change in mental status from the patient's baseline?

Did the (abnormal) behavior fluctuate during the day (ie, tend to come and go), or increase and decrease in severity?

Feature 2: Inattention

This feature is shown by a positive response to the following question: Did the patient have difficulty focusing attention (eg, being easily distractible) or having difficulty keeping track of what was being said?

Feature 3: Disorganized Thinking

This feature is shown by a positive response to the following question: Was the patient's thinking disorganized or incoherent, such as rambling or irrelevant conversation, unclear or illogical flow of ideas, or unpredictable switching from subject to subject?

Feature 4: Altered Level of Consciousness

This feature is shown by any answer other than "alert" to the following question:

Overall, how would you rate this patient's level of consciousness? (alert [normal], vigilant [hyperalert], lethargic [drowsy, easily aroused], stupor [difficult to arouse], coma [unarousable]).

The diagnosis of delirium by CAM requires the presence of features 1 and 2 and either 3 or 4.
From Inouye S, van Dyck C, Alessi C, et al. Clarifying confusion: the confusion assessment method. Ann Intern Med 1990;113(12):941–8. © 2003 Sharon K. Inouye, MD, MPH.

DIFFERENTIATING PSYCHIATRIC PRESENTATION FROM DELIRIUM

Many psychiatric patients inherently have some degree of alteration of their mental status ranging from problems with perception such as hallucinations and delusions, to problems with insight. To confound matters, anxiety, psychotic, or emotional components could be present during a delirious process. This makes the diagnosis of delirium in patients with psychiatric illness challenging and prone to errors, as care providers often erroneously attribute the changes in mental status to psychiatric illness. These patients are at risk of being overlooked due to the presumption that their behavior is likely caused by their psychiatric illness. However, this subset of patients for whom psychiatric illness alone accounts for the cause of undifferentiated altered mental status is actually relatively small, 2% to 14%, depending on the population being studied.[1,6,7]

Some medical conditions can exacerbate underlying psychiatric symptoms or precipitate a new onset of psychiatric symptoms in someone without history of mental illness. Hence the key for effective management relies on the high index of suspicion for delirium regardless of the presence of psychiatric history, identifying, stabilizing, and treating the underlying etiology.

Certain clinical factors, shown in **Table 1**, can help the emergency physician accomplish this task. Basically, patients with psychiatric cause of AMS are typically alert, oriented, and rarely have visual hallucinations.

HISTORY

Obtaining history is often challenging, because the patients themselves are often confused. However, when obtained, history can provide immense insight into the possible reasons for mental status change. In 1 study,[1] the history of present illness provided the greatest diagnostic value, providing about 51% of positive clues that led to eventual diagnosis (**Fig. 1**). Hence collateral information should be sought from previous medical records and from family members, friends, emergency medical service personnel, or other acquaintances. Valuable insights are those that address the features in **Fig. 2** and **Box 1**, as well as other clinical symptoms associated with the mental status change, such as: fever, headache, expression of suicide ideation, alcohol or recreational drug use, and falls or trauma.

It is well known that patients with an age greater than 65 or an underling cognitive impairment (such as dementia) are at an increased risk for delirium. A list of

Table 1		
Clinical factors that differentiate delirium from psychiatric illness		
Characteristics	Delirium	Psychiatric Illness
Onset	Acute[a]	Subacute or chronic[a]
Course	Fluctuation	Constant
Vital signs	Usually abnormal	Usually normal (except in acute agitation)
Orientation	Usually impaired	Rarely impaired
Attention	Impaired	Usually normal
Hallucinations	Primarily visual	Primarily auditory
Awareness	Impaired	Usually intact

[a] From patient's previous baseline level of functioning or mental status.[8]
Adapted from Sood TR, Mcstay CM. Evaluation of the psychiatric patient. Emerg Med Clin N Am 2009;27:671.

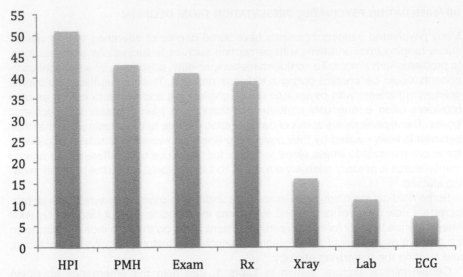

Fig. 1. Value of the various features of the diagnostic evaluation of AMS. The laboratory panel includes chemistry panel (5%), complete blood count (1%), coagulation panel (0%), and urinalysis (11%). (*Data from* Kanich W, Brady WJ, Huff JS, et al. Altered mental status: evaluation and etiology in the ED. Am J Emerg Med 2002;20(7):613–7.)

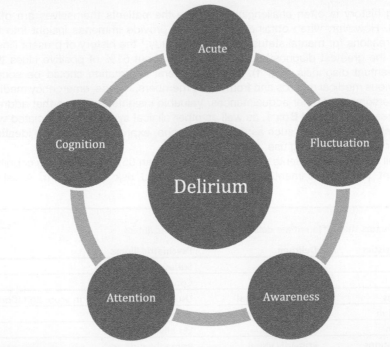

Fig. 2. Summary of key diagnostic words of delirium based on DSM-5. Disturbance in attention refers to reduced ability to direct, focus, sustain, and shift attention. Disturbance in awareness refers to reduced orientation to the environment. Disturbance in cognition refers to memory deficit, disorientation, language, visuospatial ability, or perception. Fluctuation alludes to change in symptoms during the course of a day.

medications and recent changes in medications and dosages is crucial, as polypharmacy and certain medications are known to precipitate delirium. These medications include opioids, anticholinergics, antihistamines, sedative hypnotics, and steroids.[9-11]

PHYSICAL EXAMINATION

Physical examination is a great tool that is always available to the physician and can aid with narrowing the differential diagnosis (see **Fig. 1**). Although at times challenging because of patients' agitation or uncooperativeness, a thorough physical examination that extends beyond the cardiovascular systems is indicated in all patients with AMS. Physicians should pay attention to the following:

- Head, eyes, ears, nose, throat. It is important to examine the head, as it can show signs of trauma. Poorly reactive pupils may suggest cerebral herniation. Exophthalmos may indicate underlying thyroid pathology. Eye examination can also give a clue about possible toxidromes (miosis, mydriasis, nystagmus). Other signs of toxidromes are shown in **Table 2**. Opthalmoplegia could suggest Wernicke encephalopathy in the appropriate clinical setting. Vertical nystagmus can be a sign of intracranial process or phencyclidine (PCP) ingestion, while rotary nystagmus can be a sign of ingestion of a drug of abuse such as PCP.
- Neck. Examination of the neck provides information about meningismus and goiter.
- Cardiovascular. New murmur can be seen in infective endocarditis, which in turn can cause sepsis and delirium.
- Respiratory. Abnormal lung sounds can suggest pneumonia (a common cause of delirium in the elderly).

Table 2		
Mental status effects and other signs of toxidromes		
Toxidromes	**Mental Status Effect**	**Signs**
Opiate	Sedation	Hypoventilation, decreased depth of respiration, miosis
Anticholinergic	Agitation or coma	Tachycardia, flushed and dry skin, dry mucus membranes, hyperthermia, decreased bowel sounds, urinary retention, mydriasis
Cholinergic	CNS depression	Muscarininc: salivation, lacrimation, urination, gastrointestinal distress, bronchorrhea, bradycardia, miosis Nicotinic: hypertension, tachycardia, fasciculations
Sympathomimetics	Agitation, seizures, coma	Hypertension, tachycardia, hyperthermia, diaphoresis, hyperpnea, mydriasis
Benzodiazepines/ alcohols	CNS depression	Decreased motor tone, hypotension
Hallucinogens	Excitation, agitation, hallucination, CNS depression	Tachycardia, mydriasis
Alcohol or benzodiazepine withdrawal	Excitation, agitation, hallucination, CNS depression	Tachycardia, mydriasis, diaphoresis, hypertension
Opiate withdrawal	Clear sensorium, anxiety	Yawning, piloerection, nausea, vomiting, tachycardia

- Skin. Skin examination might reveal diaphoresis as seen in overdose from sympathomimetics. Rashes or purpura can be seen in meningococcemia.
- Musculoskeletal. Consider muscular examination, as it could reveal lead-pipe rigidity as can be seen in neuroleptic malignant syndrome.
- Neurologic. Note patients Glasgow coma scale and check for focal neurologic deficits suggesting intracranial pathology. Asterixis can be seen in hepatic encephalopathy. Tremors can be seen in alcohol withdrawal and delirium tremens. Check reflexes looking for clonus as can be seen in serotonin syndrome, or hyperthyroidism.

WORK UP FOR ALTERED MENTAL STATUS

The differential diagnosis should guide work-up for AMS. Differential diagnosis for AMS is shown on **Box 2**.

STABILIZATION AND MANAGEMENT
First Steps

One should first assess and secure airway. Check for breathing and circulation and support as needed. Consider using lactated ringers for circulatory resuscitation if toxic ingestion is suspected, as normal saline can worsen acidosis.

The patient then should be placed on a monitor as airway, breathing and circulation are assessed. Obtain a full set of vital signs. In a nonagitated patient, unexplained vital sign abnormality is a red flag and suggests underlying systemic illness (**Table 3**).

Point of care glucose testing should be the first test performed on every patient with AMS as it identifies hypoglycemia, a common but easily reversible cause of mental status change. If the patient is febrile, and there is concern for meningitis, he or she should be promptly placed in droplet isolation while further evaluation continues.

Electrocardiogram (ECG) is a fast and relatively cheap diagnostic test that can be helpful in identifying cardiac causes of AMS change, especially in the elderly. Additionally, it provides baseline corrected QT for reference later if antipsychotics are used.

Laboratory Testing

Several basic tests are recommended in patients with AMS:

- A complete blood cell count should be conducted. Leukocytosis can suggest infection, although things like medications (like corticosteroids) and agitation can cause elevation in white blood count.[12] Thrombocytopenia can suggest pathologies like Thrombotic Thrombocytopenic Purpura or undiagnosed liver disease in the right clinical setting.
- A test for basic chemistry should be conducted. Electrolyte derangement like hypoglycemia, renal failure, and hypercalcemia can cause mental status change.
- A pregnancy test should be conducted in all females of childbearing age.
- Check alcohol level to rule out intoxication
- Check ammonia level and liver function tests if clinical history is unknown or known to include valproic acid use or underlying liver disease. Unexplained transaminitis may suggest acetaminophen toxicity in the right clinical setting.
- In the elderly and patients with underlying thyroid disease, checking thyroid-stimulating hormone (TSH) level can reveal possible thyroid storm or myxedema coma.

Box 2
Differential diagnosis for altered mental status

Electrolyte derangement

- Hypercalcemia
- Hypoglycemia
- Hyponatremia

Endocrine Disorder

- Thyroid storm
- Myxedema coma
- DKA
- HHS
- Addison's crisis

Toxicologic cause

- Medication overdose
- Intoxication with street drugs
- Alcohol intoxication
- Alcohol withdrawal
- Polypharmacy
- Medication adverse effects such as serotonin syndrome, NMS

Infection/Sepsis

Trauma

Infarction

- MI
- Ischemic stroke

Bleeding

- Hemorrhagic stroke
- GI bleed in a cirrhotic

Other causes

- CNS tumor
- Hepatic encephalopathy
- Hypertensive encephalopathy

Abbreviations: DKA, Diabetic ketoacidosis; GI, gastrointestinal; HHS, hyperglycemic hyperosmolar state; MI, myocardial infarction; NMS, neuroleptic malignant syndrome.

- It is recommended that human immunodeficiency virus (HIV) screening test be done in patients with new-onset AMS, as this could be an initial manifestation of central nervous system (CNS) infection from AIDS.
- If clinical history suggests, checking creatinine kinase level may be helpful, as AMS may precede or occur with other signs of certain pathologies like rhabdomyolysis or neuroleptic malignant syndrome.

Table 3
Pathologies to consider with vital sign abnormality in altered mental status

Vitals Sign Abnormality	Consider
Temperature[a]	Infection Endocrinopathy (eg, thyroid) Environmental (hyperthermia or hypothermia) Toxicology (NMS, sympathomimetics)
Respiratory rate	Toxicology (opiate or benzodiazepine overdose) DKA Sepsis Salicylate overdose
Blood pressure	Hypertensive encephalopathy Intracranial hemorrhage
Heart rate	Endocrinopathy Cardiac cause Toxicology (drugs of abuse) Infection
Hypoxia	Infection Infarction Substance overdose

[a] Rectal temperature is recommended in all patients with altered mental status, as mouth breathing could cause misrepresentation of true temperature.

- If the patient has other comorbidities and is on medications with measurable levels (example seizure medications, digoxin, valproic acid, lithium), the levels of these drugs should be checked for toxicity.
- Finally, other tests are deferred to the clinician based on patient's presentation, clinical suspicion, and judgment.

Is Head Computed Tomography Scan Indicated for All Cases of Altered Mental Status?

Head computed tomography (CT) is probably not indicated for all cases of AMS. However, the extent of its utility varies in the literature. The range of clinically significant findings in CT scans of the head for nontraumatic reasons varies between 8% and 45%[7,13] in the literature. Many sources agree that utility is higher in the elderly (**Table 4**). The decision about head imaging is up to the treating physician and is based on clinical factors. The authors recommend head imaging in certain patients such as new-onset AMS without an identifiable cause, elderly patients, patients on anticoagulation or antiplatelets, patients with other neurologic signs or symptoms or signs of trauma, and immunocompromised patients (or those with relative immunocompromised states such as alcoholics or patients on steroid treatment). Noncontrast head CT is usually sufficient in the acute setting.[14]

Lumbar Puncture

Lumbar puncture (LP) should be considered in all patients with high suspicion for delirium with fever. However, the authors recommend that in certain populations (the elderly and immunocompromised), LP be considered even in the absence of fever, as these patients may have meningitis without presenting with a fever. In a recent study, LP yielded diagnosis for AMS in 10 out of 84 afebrile elderly patients.[15] Also consider LP in cases of new-onset psychosis given the increasing prevalence of pathologies like anti-N-Methyl D-Aspartate Receptor encephalitis. Decision making about LP in other groups is up to the clinician based on clinical factors.

Table 4
Causes of altered mental status in patients ages 18 to 64 and greater than 65 years

Cause of Altered Mental Status	18–64 y, n (%)	>65 y, n (%)	P Value
Ischemic stroke	36.8	59.3	<.001
Hemorrhagic stroke	34.4	20.6	.004
Infection	11.9	25.8	<.001
Toxicologic	16.6	4	<.001
Cardiac	4.2	10.8	<.001
Psychiatric	14	3.1	<.001

Patients can have more than one cause of altered mental status.
From Leong LB, Wei Jian KH, Vasu A, et al. Identifying risk factors for an abnormal computed tomographic scan of the head among patients with altered mental status in the emergency department. Eur J Emerg Med 2010;17(4):222.

What About Urine Drug Screen?

Most urine drug screen (UDS) results are qualitative immunoassays that are based on specific cutoff concentration. Samples close to the cutoff may give negative or positive results depending on the precision of the assay and other sample conditions. Additionally, certain antibodies may cross-react with medications outside the target drug class, leading to false-positive results. Therefore care should be taken not to anchor prematurely based on result of UDS in a patient with AMS. If for example, a patient presents with miotic pupil and depressed respirations, treatment for likely opiate overdose should ensue even if UDS is negative for opiate, because not all opiates would test positive on UDS. **Table 5** shows common false negatives and positives on UDS.

Managing Agitation in the Emergency Department

An agitated patient poses a danger to himself or herself and hospital staff. Therefore the top priority in management of this patient is safety.

The patient should be temporarily placed in a safe area, and nonpharmacological intervention should be instituted first. The first recommended nonpharmacologic intervention is verbal de-escalation of the situation. Signs like changes in tone and speed of

Table 5
False positives and negatives on urine drug screen

Drug Class	False-Positives	False-Negatives
Amphetamines	Amantadine, bupropion, ranitidine, labetalol, desipramine, fluoxetine, trazodone, pseudoephrine	MDMA
Opiates	Dextromethorphan, diphenhydramine, fluoroquinolones, rifampin, quinine, poppy seed	Fentanyl, oxycodone, methadone, tramadol, propoxyphene
Phencyclidine	Dextromethorphan, ketamine, venlafaxine, tramadol, ibuprofen, meperidine, diphenhydramine	—
Cannabinoids	Dronabinol, nonsteroidal anti-inflammatory drugs, proton pump inhibitors	Visine eye drop
Benzodiazepines	Sertraline, oxaprozin	Midazolam, chlodiazepoxide, flunitrazepam

speech, irritability, pacing, and clenched fist or jaw all indicate that this method of intervention is insufficient.[16] At this juncture, physical restraint or pharmacologic intervention may be added.

In a patient with mild agitation, who is easily verbally redirected, a trial of oral atypical antipsychotics can be as efficacious as intravenous or intramuscular agents.[17] If a patient has severe agitation, and verbal de-escalation has failed, physical restraint may be used temporarily and with caution, realizing that such a patient, with minimal mental inhibition, is at increased risk for complications such as fractures, asphyxiation, and soft tissue damage as he or she continues to resist.[18]

In the management of severely agitated patients, the physician should observe certain aspects of patient presentation before using sedatives. For example, observe the patient's ability to move all extremities or ambulate, and the patient's presedation Glasgow coma scale (GCS).

Antipsychotics are the most commonly used first-line medications for treatment of delirium. Haloperidol is the most studied antipsychotic, and it is available in oral, intramuscular, and intravenous formulations. The most common dosage of haloperidol is 2 to 5 mg intramuscularly when other nonpharmacological and less restrictive methods failed. The risk of QT prolongation is small, but higher with the intravenous formulation; therefore, oral or intramuscular formulation is preferred. Benadryl is often given concurrently to minimize the risk of extrapyramidal adverse effects. Atypical or newer antipsychotics like risperidone, quetiapine, and olanzapine also have been used and have been shown to be effective.[19–21]

Benzodiazepines are at times used (in isolation or in combination with haloperidol) in the ED for management of agitated delirium. Lorazepam is the most commonly used benzodiazepine, at an initial dose of 2 mg intravascular. However, a prospective double-blind randomized controlled trial (RCT) found 5 mg of intramuscular midazolam to be superior to 2 mg intramuscular lorazepam or 5 mg intramuscular haloperidol by displaying quicker onset of control of agitation and more rapid time to arousal,[22–38] a feature that would be helpful if the initial history and physical examination were not successfully completed.

When delirium is suspected to be related to alcohol withdrawal, diazepam is the agent of choice, and in fact, antipsychotics should be avoided in that situation, as it lowers seizure threshold in this population. In the elderly, benzodiazepine use for agitation (whether in the ED or not) should be avoided except in alcohol withdrawal, as benzodiazepines have been linked to increased risk of developing delirium in this population.[9]

SUMMARY

AMS is a common but nonspecific ED presentation that can mask underlying serious pathology. Delirium is defined as an acute change in mental status from baseline with fluctuation in awareness, attention, and cognitive function, due to another medical condition, substance intoxication, or withdrawal.

Delirium is missed at high rates in the ED due to practice constraints such as time pressure, subtle presentation, or confounding clinical factors. It carries a high morbidity and mortality if missed, and there is a 90% chance that if delirium is missed in the ED, it would also be missed in the inpatient setting. As such, the emergency medicine physician should maintain a high index of suspicion for delirium in all patients with AMS; this is especially true for those with underlying medical or psychiatric illness or dementia, because atypical baseline in these patients can confound matters.

A thorough history and physical examination are indicated in all patients with AMS, as these provide the greatest diagnostic value in the management of patients AMS.

Laboratory studies, neuroimaging, and LP should be tailored to individual cases based on available history and physical examination findings.

Overall management of delirium is targeted toward treatment of the underlying cause. Options for management of agitated delirium include verbal redirection, physical restraints, and a pharmacologic approach with antipsychotics and benzodiazepines.

REFERENCES

1. Kanich W, Brady WJ, Huff JS, et al. Altered mental status: evaluation and etiology in the ED. Am J Emerg Med 2002;20(7):613–7.
2. Ely EW, Shintani A, Truman B, et al. Delirium as a predictor of mortality in mechanically ventilated patients in the intensive care unit. JAMA 2004;291(14):1753–62.
3. Thomason JW, Shintani A, Peterson JF, et al. Intensive care unit delirium is an independent predictor of longer hospital stay: a prospective analysis of 261 non-ventilated patients. Crit Care 2005;9(4):R375–81.
4. Han JH, Wilber ST. Altered mental status in older patients in the emergency department. Clin Geriatr Med 2013;29(1):101–36.
5. Han JH, Zimmerman EE, Cutler N, et al. Delirium in older emergency department patients: recognition, risk factors, and psychomotor subtypes. Acad Emerg Med 2009;16(3):193–200.
6. O'Keefe KP, Sanson TG. Elderly patients with altered mental status. Emerg Med Clin North Am 1998;16(4):701–15.
7. Leong LB, Wei Jian KH, Vasu A, et al. Identifying risk factors for an abnormal computed tomographic scan of the head among patients with altered mental status in the emergency department. Eur J Emerg Med 2010;17(4):219–23.
8. Sood TR, Mcstay CM. Evaluation of the psychiatric patient. Emerg Med Clin North Am 2009;27(4):669–83.
9. Pandharipande P, Shintani A, Peterson J, et al. Lorazepam is an independent risk factor for transitioning to delirium in intensive care unit patients. Anesthesiology 2006;104(1):21–6.
10. Inouye SK, Charpentier PA. Precipitating factors for delirium in hospitalized elderly persons. Predictive model and interrelationship with baseline vulnerability. JAMA 1996;275(11):852–7.
11. Young J, Murthy L, Westby M, et al. Diagnosis, prevention, and management of delirium: summary of NICE guidance. BMJ 2010;341:c3704.
12. Morgado JP, Monteiro CP, Matias CN, et al. Sex-based effects on immune changes induced by a maximal incremental exercise test in well-trained swimmers. J Sports Sci Med 2014;13(3):708–14.
13. Rothrock SG, Buchanan C, Green SM, et al. Cranial computed tomography in the emergency evaluation of adult patients without a recent history of head trauma: a prospective analysis. Acad Emerg Med 1997;4(7):654–61.
14. Shuaib W, Tiwana MH, Chokshi FH, et al. Utility of CT head in the acute setting: value of contrast and non-contrast studies. Ir J Med Sci 2014. [Epub ahead of print].
15. Shah K, Richard K, Edlow JA. Utility of lumbar puncture in the afebrile vs. febrile elderly patient with altered mental status: a pilot study. J Emerg Med 2007;32(1):15–8.
16. Zimbroff DL. Pharmacological control of acute agitation: focus on intramuscular preparations. CNS Drugs 2008;22(3):199–212.
17. Gault TI, Gray SM, Vilke GM, et al. Are oral medications effective in the management of acute agitation? J Emerg Med 2012;43(5):854–9.

18. Lagomasino I, Daly R, Stoudemire A. Medical assessment of patients presenting with psychiatric symptoms in the emergency setting. Psychiatr Clin North Am 1999;22(4):819–50, viii–ix.
19. Lonergan E, Britton AM, Luxenberg J, et al. Antipsychotics for delirium. Cochrane Database Syst Rev 2007;(2):CD005594.
20. Rea RS, Battistone S, Fong JJ, et al. Atypical antipsychotics versus haloperidol for treatment of delirium in acutely ill patients. Pharmacotherapy 2007;27(4):588–94.
21. Maneeton B, Maneeton N, Srisurapanont M, et al. Quetiapine versus haloperidol in the treatment of delirium: a double-blind, randomized, controlled trial. Drug Des Devel Ther 2013;7:657–67.
22. Nobay F, Simon BC, Levitt MA, et al. A prospective, double-blind, randomized trial of midazolam versus haloperidol versus lorazepam in the chemical restraint of violent and severely agitated patients. Acad Emerg Med 2004;11(7):744–9.
23. Saxena S, Lawley D. Delirium in the elderly: a clinical review. Postgrad Med J 2009;85(1006):405–13.
24. Van Munster BC, De Rooji S. Delirium: a synthesis of current knowledge. Clin Med 2014;14(5):548.
25. Koita J, Riggio S, Jagoda A. The mental status examination in emergency practice. Emerg Med Clin North Am 2010;28(3):439–51.
26. Tan I, Young N, Sindhusake DP, et al. Prospective evaluation of selected clinical criteria for cranial computed tomography in non-trauma adult patients. Emerg Med Australas 2009;21(1):43–51.
27. Rund DA, Ewing JD, Mitzel K, et al. The use of intramuscular benzodiazepines and antipsychotic agents in the treatment of acute agitation or violence in the emergency department. J Emerg Med 2006;31(3):317–24.
28. Rolland B, Debien C, Vaiva G. Treatment of agitation in the emergency department: benzodiazepines could be safer than antipsychotics in some cases of insufficient medical data. J Emerg Med 2014;46(6):830–1.
29. Battaglia J, Moss S, Rush J, et al. Haloperidol, lorazepam, or both for psychotic agitation? A multicenter, prospective, double-blind, emergency department study. Am J Emerg Med 1997;15(4):335–40.
30. Cañas F. Management of agitation in the acute psychotic patient–efficacy without excessive sedation. Eur Neuropsychopharmacol 2007;17(Suppl 2):S108–14.
31. Melanson SE. The utility of immunoassays for urine drug testing. Clin Lab Med 2012;32(3):429–47.
32. Wilber ST. Altered mental status in older emergency department patients. Emerg Med Clin North Am 2006;24(2):299–316, vi.
33. Brahm NC, Yeager LL, Fox MD, et al. Commonly prescribed medications and potential false-positive urine drug screens. Am J Health Syst Pharm 2010;67(16):1344–50.
34. Moeller KE, Lee KC, Kissack JC. Urine drug screening: practical guide for clinicians. Mayo Clin Proc 2008;83(1):66–76.
35. Ryan SA, Costello DJ, Cassidy EM, et al. Anti-NMDA receptor encephalitis: a cause of acute psychosis and catatonia. J Psychiatr Pract 2013;19:157–61.
36. Riahi-Zanjani B. False positive and false negative results in urine drug screening tests: tampering methods and specimen integrity tests. Pharmacologyonline 2014;1:102–8.
37. Wang HR, Woo YS, Bahk WM. Atypical antipsychotics in the treatment of delirium. Psychiatry Clin Neurosci 2013;67:323–31.
38. Campanelli CM. The American Geriatrics Society updated beers criteria for potentially inappropriate medication use in older adults. J Am Geriatr Soc 2012;60:616–31.

Depression and the Suicidal Patient

Dick C. Kuo, MD[a], Mina Tran, MD[a],*, Asim A. Shah, MD[b], Anu Matorin, MD[b]

KEYWORDS

- Depression • Suicide • Suicide risk • Emergency room

KEY POINTS

- The emergency department must maintain the safety of the patient and provide a thorough evaluation of the depressed or suicidal patient.
- Multiple screening tools may be used for depression, and all sources of information are important in providing a complete picture of patient symptoms and safety.
- Suicidal patients must be assessed for high risk and potentially protective factors to create the best disposition possible for the patient.
- Safety contracts have not been shown to be as effective as previously thought.
- Antidepressants may be initiated with the consultation and follow-up of a psychiatrist.

BACKGROUND AND EPIDEMIOLOGY

Depression is extremely common. The lifetime prevalence of depression is 20% to 25% in women and 7% to 12% in men.[1] In 2007, appoximately12 million visits to emergency departments (EDs) were related to mental health or substance abuse.[2] Typically associated with depressive symptoms or substance abuse, suicidal ideation and suicide attempts are also common in the ED, with approximately 650,000 patients evaluated in EDs for suicide attempts.[3] In a general hospital, depression accounts for approximately 50% of psychiatric consultations and 12% of all hospital admissions.[4] In recognition of this serious health impact, the Joint Commission established a National Patient Safety Goal (NPSG) to address this issue in 2010. This NPSG requires "behavioral health care organizations, psychiatric hospitals, and general hospitals treating individuals for emotional or behavioral disorders, to identify patients at risk for suicide."[5] Despite these numbers and the increased awareness established by the Joint Commission, depression is often underdiagnosed or missed completely in a busy ED. Often patients with

Disclosure: The authors have no financial disclosure or conflict of interest to declare.
[a] Section of Emergency Medicine, Department of Medicine, Baylor College of Medicine, One Baylor Plaza, Houston, TX 77030, USA; [b] Department of Psychiatry, Baylor College of Medicine, One Baylor Plaza - BCM350, Houston, TX 77030, USA
* Corresponding author.
E-mail address: minahanh@gmail.com

depression can present with vague somatic complaints such as fatigue, anxiety, weakness, headache, and chronic pain, leading to multiple ED visits.[6] Depression is a mental illness with considerable disability, morbidity, and mortality. It has been well documented that depression is a common comorbidity in other debilitating diseases such as heart disease, stroke, diabetes, cancer, dementia, and many others.[1,4,7,8] The elderly are particularly at risk, and depression can be misdiagnosed as early dementia.[3] An early study by Meldon and colleagues[9] found that recognition of depression by emergency physicians in geriatric patients was low, with a sensitivity of only 27.5%.

Risk factors for major depression include female gender, African American or Hispanic, younger age or older age in a nursing facility, and marital status being never married, widowed, or divorced.[10] In a survey performed in 15 countries by the World Health Organization, women were nearly twice as likely have depression,[11] and in the United States women had a prevalence of 8% to 10%, whereas the prevalence in men was only 3% to 5%.[12] African Americans and Hispanic Americans have a 4.0% and 4.3% prevalence of depression, respectively, compared with 3.1% in non-Hispanic whites.[13]

DEFINITION OF DEPRESSION

Patients with depression display disturbances in their mood, psychomotor activity, and thought processes, and vegetative disturbances (sleep, appetite, and sexual function). Strictly speaking, major depressive disorder (MDD) is described in the fifth edition of the *Diagnostic and Statistical Manual of Mental Disorders* (DSM-5) by 1 or more major depressive episodes.[14] According to DSM-5, major depressive disorder is established when 5 or more of the symptoms are listed (See 'DSM-5 Diagnostic Criteria for Major Depressive Disorder' in The diagnostic and statistical manual of mental disorders. American Psychiatric Association. 5th edition. Available at: http://www.dsm5.org/), and have been present during the same 2-week period and represent a change from previous functioning.[14] At least 1 of the symptoms must be either depressed mood most of the day, nearly every day (ie, feels sad, empty, or hopeless) or markedly diminished interest or pleasure in all, or almost all activities most of the day, nearly every day. Other symptoms include significant weight loss when not intentional, insomnia or hypersomnia, psychomotor agitation or retardation, fatigue or loss of energy, feelings of worthlessness or excessive or inappropriate guilt, diminished ability to think or concentrate or indecisiveness, or recurrent thoughts of death, suicidal ideation, or a suicide attempt or specific plan. Of note, lack of interest and depressed mood are the most important factors. Also noteworthy is that these symptoms should cause clinically significant distress or impairment in social, occupational, or other important areas of functioning. The episode is not attributable to physiologic effects of a substance or to another medical condition. The symptoms are not better explained by schizoaffective disorder, schizophrenia, schizophreniform disorders, delusional disorder, or other specified or unspecified schizophrenia spectrum. In addition, the patient should not have previously exhibited a manic episode or a hypomanic episode to distinguish it from bipolar disorder (BD).[4,14]

There are various subtypes of MDD, the more common of which include major depression with melancholy, major depression with psychotic features, and seasonal affective disorder. Major depression with melancholy is particularly notable because of its association with increased suicide rates.[15]

DIFFERENTIAL DIAGNOSIS

Other mental disorders have signs and symptoms similar to those of depression. In addition, depression often coexists with other mental illnesses, and it is important to recognize them to properly care and treat the patient. The differential diagnosis of depression is listed in **Box 1**.

BD is clinically very difficult to distinguish from depression, as most bipolar patients present with depression or no symptoms. Studies have shown that close to 60% of BD individuals are initially diagnosed as having depression.[16,17] However, the crucial information to distill from the patient is a history of manic or hypomanic episodes.

Anxiety disorders most commonly seen include posttraumatic stress disorder, generalized anxiety disorder, panic disorder, and obsessive-compulsive disorder. These conditions may coexist with depression, and the treatment of depression can also improve the symptoms of anxiety disorders.[1]

Dysthymia is similar to MDD but less severe. It is associated with chronic depressed mood and the same somatic and cognitive symptoms that occur in major depression, but only requires 2 additional symptoms in addition to depressed mood. Dysthymic patients are at increased risk for MDD.[1]

Adjustment disorder with depressed mood is the manifestation of depressive symptoms in response to identifiable stressors within 3 months of onset of the stressors. This stressor cannot be the death of a loved one, which would be more consistent with bereavement.

Somatic symptom disorders include conversion, body dysmorphic syndrome, hypochondriasis, and somatoform pain disorder. These disorders may also improve with treatment of coexisting depression, as 50% of unexplained pain complaints have underlying depression.[1,4]

Personality disorders are characterized by unstable relationships and self-destructive behaviors, and can often be misdiagnosed as depression. Borderline personality disorder (BPD) commonly coexists with MDD, as many patients with BPD often present with depressive symptoms,[18] and it can be difficult to distinguish between the two.

Dementia is often difficult to distinguish from depression, especially in its early stages. Dementia is characterized by abnormal mental status, memory, and judgment.

Box 1
Differential diagnosis for depression

Bipolar disorder

Anxiety disorders (posttraumatic stress disorder, generalized anxiety, panic disorder, obsessive-compulsive disorder)

Dysthymia

Adjustment disorder with depressed mood

Bereavement

Somatic symptom disorders (conversion, body dysmorphic, hypochondriasis, somatoform pain disorder)

Personality disorders (borderline personality disorder)

Dementia

Substance abuse

Depressive disorder not otherwise specified

Depression attributable to general medical conditions

Substance abuse can often present with major depression.[1,7] It is important to screen all patients with major depression for concomitant substance use, especially alcohol. Appropriate referrals can be made when necessary.

Depressive disorder not otherwise specified is a classification for patients who do not meet any of the criteria for the aforementioned mood disorders.

Depression arising from a general medical condition and medications is a broad term that includes depression caused by a medical illness such as thyroid disease (hypothyroidism or hyperthyroidism), stroke, heart disease, human immunodeficiency virus/AIDS, dementia, diabetes, cancer, medications, and many others (**Table 1**). It is estimated that 10% to 15% of all depression is due to organic causes.

ROLE OF EMERGENCY DEPARTMENT PHYSICIAN IN EVALUATING PATIENTS WITH DEPRESSION

The depressed patient has a wide potential spectrum of presentations, and may exhibit subtle somatoform complaints or present after attempting suicide. The role of the ED physician always begins with stabilization of the patient and maintaining the safety of the patient and the ED. Patient safety may include removal of any potential means of self-harm, isolation, one-to-one observation, and physical restraints or medications to control agitation and aggressive behavior. A rapid and systematic assessment should include a complete history and physical examination. Certain laboratory tests, although typically not necessary for the evaluation of a depressed patient, may be helpful in certain situations, especially if other medical conditions are present that may contribute to or mimic depression. Included in the differential for depression are many medical diseases associated with depression (see **Table 1**), and specific laboratory testing such as thyroid-stimulating hormone, folate, and vitamin B_{12} levels can be ordered if depression is suspected after completion of history and physical.

Routinely many EDs will order a complete blood count, basic metabolic profile, blood alcohol level, urinalysis, urine pregnancy test if female, and urine drug screen as part of the initial evaluation, but laboratory testing rarely changes management or disposition, and is not routinely recommended in cooperative patients who are awake and alert with normal vital signs and noncontributory medical histories.[19]

Table 1
Medical conditions associated with depression

Endocrine	Neurologic	Infectious Diseases	Nutritional Deficiency	Other
Hypothyroidism	Alzheimer	Meningitis	Thiamine (B_1)	Lupus
Addison	Huntington	Encephalitis	Pyridoxine (B_6)	Steroids
Cushing	Multiple sclerosis	Human immunodeficiency virus	Folic acid (B_9)	β-Blockers
Hyperparathyroidism	Traumatic brain injury	Lyme disease	Cobalamins (B_{12})	Ca-channel blockers
	Parkinson	—	—	Hormonal therapy
	Normal pressure hydrocephalus	—	—	Obstructive sleep apnea
	Brain mass	—	—	—

Ultimately the role of the emergency physician is to provide medical clearance and obtain psychiatric specialty evaluation if available. Details on the scope of medical clearance are discussed below. In many instances psychiatric specialty evaluation is not readily available, and the emergency physician will be responsible for a reasonable evaluation that also includes screening for suicide risk. Assessment for suicide risk is one of the most important determinations that will be made in the ED. Evaluation of all depressed patients including those who have not expressed suicidal thoughts is important. There is no direct correlation between direct questioning about suicide and increased suicidal behavior.[20] If patients are not deemed to be a suicide risk, the ED should provide resources for potential treatment and recovery.

THE EMERGENCY DEPARTMENT INTERVIEW OF DEPRESSED PATIENTS

When dealing with a depressed patient in the ED, the physician must remember that the priority is the patient. A safe and stable environment must be created for patients to discuss their concerns. It is important that when a depressed mood is detected, a physician should respond in a caring and empathetic manner whereby a rapport can be built with the patient. One should avoid leading questions and approach the patient with open-ended questions such as "I see that you seem stressed out, do you want to share what's been going on?" This approach allows patients to discuss what is troubling them. The ED physician must be able to gather as much information about the patient as possible to assess whether the patient warrants psychiatric consultation or further psychiatric evaluation. Therefore, the focus should be on questions regarding anhedonia ("what are the things you enjoy doing? Do you still do them?"), depressed mood ("have you been feeling down and blue lately?"), and suicide ("Have you felt so hopeless that you think about ending your own life? Do you have a plan?"). Many tools can be used to assess patients for depression, some of which are more useful in the ED than others.

THE ROLE OF COLLATERAL AND FAMILY SUPPORT

Family collateral is an integral part of the interview with the depressed patient. Depressed patients may have poor insight into their own conditions or may not want to be forthcoming with their symptoms; therefore, collateral information must be obtained for the physician to make an appropriate assessment and evaluation. Information obtained from a collateral source is especially important when patients are not able to detail their own symptoms.[21] Knowing a patient's family support also helps the physician understand the patient's situation, and is an important factor in deciding patient disposition. Studies have revealed that less supportive and more conflicting family environments are associated with greater depressive symptomatology.[22]

SCREENING TOOLS FOR DEPRESSION

Probably one of the easiest ways to remember the symptoms for depression is the mnemonic SIG E CAPS[23] (**Box 2**). Patients with any of these symptoms should likely be investigated further. Screening tools that may help include the Beck Depression Inventory,[24] the Geriatric Depression Inventory,[25,26] and the Patient Health Questionnaire (PHQ)-9.[27] PHQ-9 is a screening instrument that consists of 9 questions that assess the patient for symptoms of depression as characterized in the DSM-5 for MDD, and is outlined in **Box 3**. There is also the PHQ-2, which shows similar sensitivity

---

Box 2
The mnemonic SIG E CAPS

Sleep amount (either increased or decreased)

Interest (anhedonia)

Guilt

Energy level decreased

Concentration decreased

Appetite (either increased or decreased)

Psychomotor activity (either increased or decreased)

Suicidal ideation

---

and specificity for the detection of depression[28] while only using 2 major symptoms of decreased interest in daily activities and depressed mood.

The original Geriatric Depression Scale was a 30-item questionnaire used in patients aged 65 and older. It has been validated in younger adults and there is also a 15-item and 5-question version.[26,29] Biros and colleagues[30] have also used the Beck Depression Inventory in the ED population to examine the incidence of depression.

Box 3
Patient health questionnaire 9 (PHQ-9)

Patient fills out questionnaire that asks "Over the last 2 weeks, have you had the following problems?" The patient is asked to respond "not at all" (0 points), "several days" (1 point), "more than half the days" (2 points), "nearly every day" (3 points).

1. Little interest or pleasure in doing things

2. Feeling down, depressed, or hopeless

3. Trouble falling or staying asleep or sleeping too much

4. Feeling tired or having little energy

5. Poor appetite or overeating

6. Feeling bad about yourself or that you are a failure or have let yourself or your family down

7. Trouble concentrating on things, such as reading the newspaper or watching television

8. Moving or speaking so slowly that other people have noticed, or the opposite, being so fidgety or restless that you have been moving around a lot more

9. Thought you would be better off dead, or of hurting yourself in some way

Total Score

1–4: minimal depression

5–9: mild depression

10–14: moderate depression

15–19: moderately severe depression

20–27: severe depression

ASSESSMENT OF SUICIDE
Suicidality

Patients in a depressed state often feel so profoundly worthless and hopeless that they contemplate taking their own life. Suicide assessment must be done in all patients with depression, as suicide is one of the top 10 leading causes of death in all age groups.[1] Patients who present to the ED with deliberate self-harm are at 6-fold higher risk for eventually completing suicide, and at least 15% of patients with recurrent depression will eventually kill themselves.[31,32] Ajdacic-Gross and colleagues[33] showed that the suicide risk for psychiatric inpatients is about 50 times higher than for the general population.[34]

Mental health professionals distinguish 5 categories of suicide (**Table 2**), namely completed suicide, suicide attempt, suicide gesture, suicide gamble, and suicidal ideation, with the latter being the most common.[35]

Methods of Suicide

There are many different methods of self-harm, of which death from firearms accounts for the majority. As noted previously, the major predictor of successful suicide is previous attempts. Previously attempted methods that pose the highest risks for later completed suicide are hanging, strangulation, and suffocation, following by drowning, jumping, and shooting. The most lethal form of suicide is use of firearms, followed by hanging.[36,37]

Suicide Risk Factors and Assessment: High Versus Low/Moderate Risk

The purpose of suicide risk assessment is to identify high risk and protective factors.[38] Suicide risk factors are listed in **Table 3**. Of note, the best predictor of completed suicide is a history of previous attempts, and individuals, especially those with psychosis, who attempt to kill themselves by hanging, drowning, shooting, or jumping are at extremely high risk for completed suicide.[36] Given the high stakes associated with suicide, obtaining an accurate suicide risk assessment is critical to the patient's treatment and management. Although not standardized, the spectrum of suicide risk can be viewed along a timeline: imminent, near-term, and long-term risk. A good ED physician should be able to screen for patients who are at imminent risk for suicide. This approach includes detecting when clinically actionable risk is present, identifying when an individual requires immediate attention to guarantee safety, and obtaining appropriate mental health consultation for further assessment.[39] Risk assessment is

Table 2 Types of suicide	
Type of Suicidal Behavior	**Description**
Completed suicide	The act of taking one's own life, results in death
Suicide attempt	The unsuccessful act of taking one's own life or engagement of self-injurious behavior with some intent to die
Suicide gesture	Acting out behavior, not necessarily lethal, usually low level of intent or planning to die
Suicide gamble	Behavior whereby one takes the risk that he or she will be discovered in time and that the discoverer will save them
Suicidal ideation	Thinking about suicide

Data from Brent D, Willingham E, Frey R. Suicide. The Gale encyclopedia of medicine. vol. 5. 4th edition. Detroit (MI): Gale; 2011. p. 4203–10.

Table 3
Factors that increase the risk of suicide

Risk Factors for Suicide	
Demographic	
Male sex	Caucasian race
Age >75 y	—
History	
Family history of suicide	Previous suicide attempts
History of child abuse or traumatic childhood experience	Recent stressful life event (divorce, job loss)
Medical History	
Chronic pain or illness or severe or intractable pain	Loss of mobility of independence
Alcohol or substance abuse	Presence of psychiatric illness
High cholesterol	—
Method of Suicide	
Hanging	Drowning
By firearm	Jumping from height
Lethal overdose	Walking in front of busy traffic
Worrisome Recent Behaviors	
Sudden interest in reading books/articles on death or suicide	Talking a lot about death or suicide or expressing hopelessness
Stockpiling of medications or increase intake of prescription medications	Giving away cherished possessions, writing long letters or elaborate farewells
New interest in firearms	Revising a will suddenly
Disrupted sleep pattern or refusing to take care of oneself	Increase intake of alcohol

Data from Brent D, Willingham E, Frey R. Suicide. The Gale encyclopedia of medicine. vol. 5. 4th edition. Detroit (MI): Gale; 2011. p. 4203–10; and Baylor College of Medicine Emergency Psychiatry Group, unpublished data, 2014.

a thought-provoking process that must document the analysis of the patient's overall condition and risk factors. Lower-risk situations should also be documented. Lower-risk behaviors include cutting the wrist (especially superficial cuts with no requirement of sutures), low-acuity overdose on medications, and walking out into traffic a low-volume street. Recognition of or insight into bad decision making and future orientation have also been listed as lower-risk situations. All available collateral information should be obtained to make the best assessment possible using all supporting information.

Suicide Protective Factors

It is arguably as important to assess protective risk factors as it is to assess risk factors for suicide, as the assessment of both can lead to a better evaluation of a patient's actual suicide risk.[40] Omission of a patient's protective risk factors may lead the physician to overestimate a patient's suicide risk, whereas failure to acknowledge a patient's lack of protective factors may lead to underestimation of his or her suicide risk. Protective factors that lower the risk of suicide are listed in **Box 4** and include a network of friendship, religious faith, and practice that especially discourages suicide, a stable marriage or intimate relationship, pregnancy, closely knit extended family, and a strong interest in the community or project that brings people together.

Suicide Prevention Contract and Lack of Effectiveness

It was initially thought that drawing up a suicide prevention contract would act as a protective measure, but studies have shown that suicide prevention contracts do not prevent suicide.[40] The suicide prevention contract, also known as the No Harm Contract, has been used widely, although there has been no broad consensus regarding its value, efficacy, and validity.[41,42] In fact, suicide safety contracts can be easily challenged in the courts and show no added benefits, and have been used against physicians.

SAD PERSONS

In 1983 the SAD PERSONS scale (SPS) was developed by Patterson and colleagues,[43] who found it to be useful in helping to disposition patients at risk for suicide. In 1988, Hockberger and Rothstein[44] studied the SAD PERSONS scale in ED patients in southern California, and developed a modified SAD PERSONS scale (MSPS). Comparison of the 2 scales is shown in **Table 4**. Higher scores are correlated with increased incidence of hospitalization when compared with the gold standard of qualified psychiatrist evaluation. As one of the few quick and simple evaluation tools available, the SAD PERSONS scale has gained widespread use in clinical and educational settings. However, a recent systematic review of SAD PERSONS highlighted the overall lack of literature evaluating the scale and the high variability in the outcome measures of those studies that did exist.[45] Only 3 studies[46–48] have looked at the hard outcome measure of actually predicting suicide, and these systematic reviews concluded that the SPS could not be used to predict suicidal behavior. The assessment of studies evaluating the MSPS was mixed, but current evidence also does not support its use in predicting suicidal behavior. Ultimately more studies are needed to assess the defined outcomes of future suicide and suicide risk.

DISPOSITION IN THE EMERGENCY DEPARTMENT
Access to Specialist or Psychiatric Hospitalization

In many hospitals a separate psychiatric unit is held within the ED to admit patients with acute psychiatric illnesses and emergencies. The role of the ED physician is to facilitate

Table 4
SAD PERSONS (0–2, send home with follow-up; 3–4, close follow-up, consider hospitalization; 5–6, strongly consider hospitalization depending on confidence in the follow-up arrangement; 7–10, hospitalize or commit) versus modified SAD PERSONS (MSPS)

	SAD PERSONS (1 pt Each)	MSPS (Weighted for Factors with High Significance)
S	Sex (male)	Sex (male) (1 pt)
A	Age (<19 or >45)	Age (<19 or >45) (1 pt)
D	Depression	Depression or hopelessness (2 pts)
P	Previous suicide attempt	Previous attempts or psychiatric care (previous inpatient or outpatient psychiatric care) (1 pt)
E	Ethanol abuse	Excessive alcohol or drug use (1 pt)
R	Rational thinking loss	Rational thinking loss (2 pts)
S	Social supports lacking	Separated, divorced, or widowed (1 pt)
O	Organized plan	Organized or serious attempt (2 pts)
N	No spouse	No social supports (1 pt)
S	Sickness	Stated future intent (determined to repeat attempt or ambivalent) (2 pts)

Modified weighted score found hospital discharge frequent in patients with score ≤5; patients with score 6–8 required emergent psychiatric evaluation; patients with score ≤9 were all hospitalized.

Abbreviation: pt(s), patient(s).

and coordinate care with psychiatry staff. Communication between the ED physician and the psychiatric staff is critical. Once a patient is medically cleared by the ED physician the patient is ready for psychiatric evaluation, although in many circumstances cooperative patients with normal vital signs may be evaluated before or simultaneously with "medical clearance." Depending on the severity of the condition, a patient may require inpatient admission as opposed to initiation or modification of certain medications. Suicide prevention strategies include pharmacotherapy, psychotherapy, and development of safety plans.[49] Many hospitals also have other ancillary services in addition to psychiatric services that will help depressed patients in their process of recovery. These services include social work (housing, financial, and transportation hardships), substance abuse referrals, and group therapy. However, not every hospital will have a separate psychiatric emergency room or in-house specialist. In such cases, the ED physician must make the decision of whether it is safe to discharge the patient, or whether admission and continued psychiatric evaluation and care is necessary.

When to Admit

Patients who are a danger to themselves or others will require admission to the hospital. Many of the factors already discussed will contribute to the decision-making process. All potential risk and protective factors will be considered and weighed against the patient's presentation and history. Ultimately if there is a concern that the patient is unable to be kept safe, admission for further monitoring is warranted. Involuntary restraint of the patient may be required for actively suicidal or psychotic patients with depressed mood. Admission should also be considered for patients with severe depression without active suicidal ideation, potentially on an involuntary basis.

When to Discharge

Patients can be discharged if they are deemed at low risk for self-harm. It is important to obtain collateral information from friends and family. Low-risk patients with strong family support are also potentially good candidates for discharge, especially if psychiatric follow-up can be scheduled in an appropriate time frame. When patients are deemed suitable for discharge from the ED, a systematic discharge tool, such as a checklist, should be used to ensure adequate discharge assessment and instructions. This checklist should include medications, activities of daily living, mental health follow-up, residence, follow-up psychiatric health care, and special education, financial, and other needs.[50] Medications given to newly discharged patients (including antidepressants if initiated) should be documented, including medication instructions and dosage. Compliance should be emphasized to patients and family members, as a frequent cause of readmission is medication noncompliance.[51] Follow-up with a psychiatrist or specialist in mental health is also required when patients are discharged from the ED to ensure continuity of psychiatric care and monitoring of medication efficacy. Equally important should be follow-up with medical care, as medical illness has been shown to be more frequent among patients with mental illness than in the general population.[50] The patient's social situation also helps the physician decide how much support and supervision a patient will need after discharge. A patient living alone may need more counseling before discharge in comparison with a patient living in a community home or with family who are in tune to the patient's needs. Other special considerations include financial assistance, transportation, or assistance in obtaining follow-up care. Coordination of social services is of great benefit to patients.

When to Initiate Antidepressants in the Emergency Department

Typically, antidepressant medications are not initiated by an emergency physician. Today, with an increasing number of patients receiving initial assessment in the psychiatric emergency setting and the availability of safer medications, antidepressant medications can be safely initiated in the ED[32] as part of a comprehensive care plan. However, antidepressant medication should only be initiated with psychiatric consultation and follow-up. When deciding to administer an antidepressant the selection of a specific antidepressant is based on the medication's efficacy, side-effect and safety profile, ease of administration, and cost to the patient, and on the patient's medical and family history of response. The patient and family must be educated about medication compliance. In addition to decreasing readmission, medication adherence has also been shown to decrease the rate of relapse.[52]

Relationship Between Antidepressant Initiation and Suicide Risk

In 2004, the Food and Drug Administration placed a black-box warning on all antidepressants because of concerns that such medications increase the risk of suicidal thoughts and behavior in youth; in 2006, the warning was extended to include young adults up to age 26 years. Data show that antidepressants seem to protect against suicidal events in adults. Antidepressants are effective in reducing symptoms, which, in turn, mediates suicidal events in adults and the elderly. In youth, antidepressant medications can reduce the severity of depression but seem to have no effect one way or the other on suicidal thoughts and behavior.[53,54]

SUMMARY

Depression and suicidal thoughts are a frequent presentation in the ED. The safety of the patient must be maintained while a complete and thorough evaluation is performed. Suicidal patients need to be assessed for high-risk and potential protective factors. In high-risk patients or patients for whom there remains concern for safety, psychiatric consultation or inpatient evaluation should be initiated, and involuntary restraint of the patient may be necessary. A coordinated care plan is the best option for the patient, whether inpatient or outpatient.

REFERENCES

1. Feldman MD, Christensen JF. Behavioral medicine: a guide for clinical practice. 4th edition. New York: McGraw-Hill Medical; 2014.
2. Owens P, Mutter R, Stocks C. Mental health and substance abuse-related emergency department visits among adults, 2007. Statistical Brief, Healthcare Cost and Utilization Project 2010. Rockville (MD): Agency for Healthcare Research and Quality. Available at: http://www.hcup-us.ahrq.gov/reports/statbriefs/sb92. pdf.
3. Spicer RS, Miller TR. Suicide acts in 8 states: incidence and case fatality rates by demographics and method. Am J Public Health 2000;90(12):1885–91.
4. Ropper A, Adams R, Victor M, et al. Depression and bipolar disease. Adams and Victor's principles of neurology. 10th edition. New York: McGraw-Hill Medical; 2014.
5. The Joint Commission. A follow-up report on preventing suicide: focus on medical/surgical units and the emergency department. Sentinel Event Alert 2010;46: 1–4.
6. Simms LJ, Prisciandaro JJ, Krueger RF, et al. The structure of depression, anxiety and somatic symptoms in primary care. Psychol Med 2012;42(1):15–28.
7. Kane RL. Diagnosis and management of depression. Essentials of clinical geriatrics. New York: McGraw-Hill Medical; 2013.
8. Guthrie EA, Dickens C, Blakemore A, et al. Depression predicts future emergency hospital admissions in primary care patients with chronic physical illness. J Psychosom Res 2014, in press.
9. Meldon SW, Emerman CL, Schubert DS. Recognition of depression in geriatric ED patients by emergency physicians. Ann Emerg Med 1997;30(4):442–7.
10. Chang B, Gitlin D, Patel R. The depressed patient and suicidal patient in the emergency department: evidence-based management and treatment strategies. Emerg Med Pract 2011;13(9):1–23.
11. Seedat S, Scott KM, Angermeyer MC, et al. Cross-national associations between gender and mental disorders in the World Health Organization World Mental Health Surveys. Arch Gen Psychiatry 2009;66(7):785–95.
12. Kessler RC, Chiu W, Demler O, et al. Prevalence, severity, and comorbidity of 12-month DSM-IV disorders in the national comorbidity survey replication. Arch Gen Psychiatry 2005;62(6):617–27.
13. Centers for Disease Control and Prevention (CDC). Current depression among adults—United States, 2006 and 2008. MMWR Morb Mortal Wkly Rep 2010; 59(38):1229–35.
14. American Psychiatric Association, DSM-5 Task Force. Major depression disorder: DSM-5. Washington, DC: American Psychiatric Association; 2013. p. 160–88.
15. Bradvik L, Berglund M. Repetition of suicide attempts across episodes of severe depression. Behavioural sensitisation found in suicide group but not in controls. BMC Psychiatry 2011;11:5.
16. Hirschfeld RM, Lewis L, Vornik LA. Perceptions and impact of bipolar disorder: how far have we really come? Results of the national depressive and manic-depressive association 2000 survey of individuals with bipolar disorder. J Clin Psychiatry 2003;64:161–74.

17. Goodwin FK, Jamison KR, Ghaemi SN. Manic-depressive illness: bipolar disorders and recurrent depression. New York: Oxford University Press; 2007.
18. Beatson JA, Rao S. Depression and borderline personality disorder. Med J Aust 2013;199:S24.
19. Lukens TW, Wolf SJ, Edlow JA, et al. Clinical policy: critical issues in the diagnosis and management of the adult psychiatric patient in the emergency department. Ann Emerg Med 2006;47(1):79–99.
20. Deeley ST, Love AW. Does asking adolescents about suicidal ideation induce negative mood state? Violence Vict 2010;25(5):677–88.
21. Chang YP, Edwards DF, Lach HW. The Collateral Source version of the Geriatric Depression Scale: evaluation of psychometric properties and discrepancy between collateral sources and patients with dementia in reporting depression. Int Psychogeriatr 2011;23:961–8.
22. Sheeber L, Hops H, Alpert A, et al. Family support and conflict: prospective relations to adolescent depression. J Abnorm Child Psychol 1997;25(4):333–44.
23. Rosen P, Marx J, Hockberger R, et al. Mood disorders. Rosen's emergency medicine concepts and clinical practice. Philadelphia: Mosby/Elsevier; 2014.
24. Beck AT, Ward CH, Mendelson M, et al. An inventory for measuring depression. Arch Gen Psychiatry 1961;4:561–71.
25. Yesavage JA, Sheikh JI. Geriatric Depression Scale (GDS). Clin Gerontol 1986; 5(1–2):165–73.
26. Rule BG, Harvey HZ, Dobbs AR. Reliability of the geriatric depression scale for younger adults. Clinical Gerontologist 1990;9(2):37–43.
27. Gilbody S, Richards D, Brealey S, et al. Screening for depression in medical settings with the Patient Health Questionnaire (PHQ): a diagnostic meta-analysis. J Gen Intern Med 2007;22(11):1596–602.
28. Corson K, Gerrity M, Dobscha SK. Screening for depression and suicidality in a VA primary care setting: 2 items are better than 1 item. Am J Manag Care 2004; 10(11):839–54.
29. Rinaldi P, Mecocci P, Benedetti C, et al. Validation of the five-item geriatric depression scale in elderly subjects in three different settings. J Am Geriatr Soc 2003;51(5):694–8.
30. Biros MH, Mann J, Hanson R, et al. Unsuspected or unacknowledged depressive symptoms in young adult emergency department patients. Acad Emerg Med 2009;16(4):288–94.
31. Simel DL, Rennie D, Keitz SA. Update: depression. The rational clinical examination: evidence-based clinical diagnosis. New York: McGraw-Hill; 2009.
32. Glick R. Initiation of antidepressant medications in the emergency setting. Psychiatr Ann 2000;30(4):251–7.
33. Ajdacic-Gross V, Lauber C, Baumgartner M, et al. In-patient suicide—a 13-year assessment. Acta Psychiatr Scand 2009;120:71–5.
34. Lin SK, I lung TM, Liao YT, et al. Protective and risk factors for inpatient suicides: a nested case-control study. Psychiatry Res 2014;217(1–2):54–9.
35. Brent D, Willingham E, Frey R. 4th edition. Suicide. The Gale encyclopedia of medicine, vol. 5. Detroit (MI): Gale; 2011. p. 4203–10.
36. Runeson B, Tidemalm D, Dahlin M, et al. Method of attempted suicide as predictor of subsequent successful suicide: national long term cohort study. BMJ 2010; 341:c3222.
37. Elnour AA, Harrison J. Lethality of suicide methods. Inj Prev 2008;14(1):39–45.
38. Simon RI. Improving suicide risk assessment. Psychiatr Times 2011;28(11): 16–21.

39. Boudreaux ED, Horowitz LM. Suicide risk screening and assessment: designing instruments with dissemination in mind. Am J Prev Med 2014;47(3 Suppl 2):S163–9.

40. Simon R. Assessing protective factors against suicide: questioning assumptions. Psychiatr Times 2011;28(8):35–7.

41. Stanford EJ, Goetz RR, Bloom JD. The No Harm Contract in the emergency assessment of suicidal risk. J Clin Psychiatry 1994;55:344–8.

42. Edwards SJ, Sachmann MD. No-suicide contracts, no-suicide agreements, and no-suicide assurances: a study of their nature, utilization, perceived effectiveness, and potential to cause harm. Crisis 2010;31:290–302.

43. Patterson WM, Dohn HH, Bird J, et al. Evaluation of suicidal patients: the SAD PERSONS scale. Psychosomatics 1983;24(4):343–5, 348–9.

44. Hockberger RS, Rothstein RJ. Assessment of suicide potential by nonpsychiatrists using the SAD PERSONS score. J Emerg Med 1988;6(2):99–107.

45. Warden S, Spiwak R, Sareen J, et al. The SAD PERSONS scale for suicide risk assessment: a systematic review. Arch Suicide Res 2014;18(4):313–26.

46. Ryan J, Rushdy A, Perez-Avila C, et al. Suicide rate following attendance at an accident and emergency department with deliberate self harm. Emerg Med J 1996;13:101–4.

47. Kurz A, Moller H, Torhorst A, et al. Validation of six risk scales for suicide attempters. Current Issues of Suicidology 1988;174–8.

48. Bolton JM, Spiwak R, Sareen J. Predicting suicide attempts with the SAD PERSONS scale: a longitudinal analysis. J Clin Psychiatry 2012;73:e735–41.

49. Soriano R. Depression, dementia, and delirium. New York: Springer; 2007.

50. Hochberger JM. A discharge check list for psychiatric patients. J Psychosoc Nurs Ment Health Serv 1995;33(12):35–8.

51. Libermanm RP, Massel HK, Mosk MD, et al. Social skills training for chronic mental patients. Hosp Community Psychiatry 1985;36:396–403.

52. Keene M. Confusion and complaints: the true cost of noncompliance in antidepressant therapy. Medscape Psychiatry and Health 2005;10(2). Available at: http://www.medscape.org/viewarticle/518273.

53. Gibbons RD, Hur K, Brown CH, et al. Benefits from antidepressants: synthesis of 6-week patient-level outcomes from double-blind placebo-controlled randomized trials of fluoxetine and venlafaxine. Arch Gen Psychiatry 2012;69(6):572–9.

54. Gibbons RD, Brown CH, Hur K, et al. Suicidal thoughts and behavior with antidepressant treatment: reanalysis of the randomized placebo-controlled studies of fluoxetine and venlafaxine. Arch Gen Psychiatry 2012;69(6):580–7.

New Drugs of Abuse and Withdrawal Syndromes

Sara Andrabi, MD[a],*, Spencer Greene, MD, MS[a], Nidal Moukkadam, MD, PhD[b],
Benjamin Li, MD[c]

KEYWORDS

• NBOMe • Amphetamine • Synthetic cannabinoid • Drug withdrawal • Drug abuse

KEY POINTS

• New drugs of abuse are emerging at an exponential rate. As law enforcement attempts to ban these legal highs, new chemicals are used to replace those that are prohibited.

• Newer drugs, such as NBOMe, synthetic cannabinoids, share mechanisms of action with already existing drug classes but can have atypical or severe clinical presentations.

• It is important to recognize substance use disorders when they are encountered in the emergency department. Careful consideration should be given about how to approach the patient with substance use disorder so that they can be transitioned to the appropriate outpatient treatment.

• The first priority when evaluating a patient with suspected intoxication is ensuring safety of staff and other patients, after which one should ensure the patient has a protected airway.

• Management is guided by the patient's symptoms, and basic laboratory test results, including creatinine levels, complete blood count (CBC), and liver function tests, can help diagnose end-organ damage. Midazolam may be the fastest therapeutic option to sedate patients.

NBOMe

A new group of phenethylamine derivatives called NBOMe have gained popularity among new drugs of abuse. These are phenethylamine derivatives of the 2C class of hallucinogens and include 25I-NBOMe, 25C-NBOMe, and 25B-NBOMe.[1–3] One of the most common within the NBOMe group is 25I-NBOMe, which has emerged in the designer drug market as a legal replacement for lysergic acid diethylamide

Disclosure Statement: The authors have nothing to disclose.
[a] Section of Emergency Medicine, Emergency Center, Baylor College of Medicine, 1504 Taub Loop, Houston, TX 77030, USA; [b] Stabilization, Treatment and Rehabilitation (STAR) Program for Psychosis, Menninger Department of Psychiatry, Baylor College of Medicine, 1504 Taub Loop, Houston, TX 77030, USA; [c] Menninger Department of Psychiatry, Harris Health System, Baylor College of Medicine, 1504 Taub Loop, Houston, TX 77030, USA
* Corresponding author.
E-mail address: andrabi.sara@gmail.com

Emerg Med Clin N Am 33 (2015) 779–795
http://dx.doi.org/10.1016/j.emc.2015.07.006
0733-8627/15/$ – see front matter Published by Elsevier Inc.

emed.theclinics.com

(LSD) or even sold as LSD in the illicit drug market. It is referred to by street names, including BOM-Cl, INBMeO, Holland Film, Legal Acid, N-Bomb, N-boom, NE-BOME, Smiles, Solaris, and 25-I.[4]

25I-NBOMe is the most common of the synthetic derivatives of the classical serotonergic hallucinogen 2C-I. Both are shown in **Fig. 1** for comparison. This name comes from the *N*-benzylmethoxy substituent.[5] The chemical shorthand for methoxy is OMe. Functional activity studies suggest that 25I-NBOMe is a full agonist at the 5-hydroxytryptamine (5-HT) 2A receptor. The addition of the *N*-2-methoxybenzyl group has been shown to increase binding affinity and potency when compared with 2C-I. Stimulation of this receptor is essential for the hallucinogenic effects described for drugs such as NBOMe and LSD.[6,7] The hallucinogenic effects of 25I-NBOMe have been studied in mice by observing head-twitch behavioral response (HTR). HTR functions as a surrogate marker of the hallucinogenic effect of 5-HT_{2A} receptor activation in humans.[8] This study found that 25I-NBOMe induces HTR in mice that is dose dependent and significant when compared with controls.[9]

The routes of administration for 25I-NBOMe may include sublingual, buccal (especially blotter paper; **Fig. 2**), nasal (insufflation and absorption of liquid solutions), oral, injection (intravenous and intramuscular), rectal, and inhalation.[3] The available information suggests that a range of doses are used, which in part depends on the route of administration. Blotters are the most noted method of administration, and doses may range from high microgram to low milligram levels. LSD is commonly taken sublingually in form of blotters and is one of the reasons that 25I-NBOMe is marketed as LSD in the drug market.[10]

The NBOMe compounds are highly potent 5HT_{2A} receptor agonists and α-adrenergic receptor agonists, accounting for their serotonergic and sympathomimetic symptoms. The 5-HT_{2A} receptor has been closely linked to behaviors including working memory, cognitive processes, and affective disorders such as schizophrenia. These receptors are believed to mediate the primary effects of hallucinogenic drugs such as 25I-NBOMe. Given the relationship at the 5-HT_{2A} receptor, there is concern for potential interaction with other substances that act on the serotonergic system, such as selective serotonin reuptake inhibitors and serotonin and norepinephrine (NE) reuptake inhibitors. Symptoms such as tachycardia, hypertension, hyperthermia, muscle rigidity, and convulsions should be monitored, as development of serotonergic toxicity can be a possibility in these patients. **Table 1** lists various effects noted with the drug.[3,4,11,12] The detection of 25I-NBOMe has been shown by gas chromatography and liquid chromatography coupled with mass spectrometry.[13,14]

Fig. 1. Molecular structures of 25I-NBOMe and 2C-I. (*From* EMCDDA-Europol. EMCDDA–Europol Joint Report on a New Psychoactive Substance: 25I-NBOMe. 2014. Available at: http://www.emcdda.europa.eu/. Accessed March 27, 2014.)

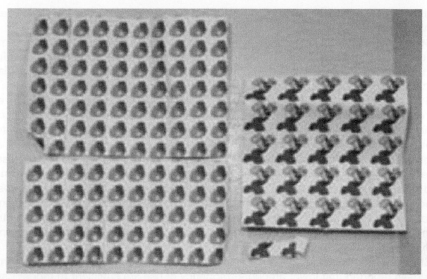

Fig. 2. Blotter paper. (*From* EMCDDA-Europol. EMCDDA–Europol Joint Report on a New Psychoactive Substance: 25I-NBOMe. 2014. Available at: http://www.emcdda.europa.eu/. Accessed March 27, 2014.)

STIMULANTS

Stimulants refer to any substance that enhances focus and may also elevate mood, improve wakefulness, and decrease appetite. The most common stimulants are nicotine, methylxanthines, and amphetamines. Milder stimulants such as methylphenidate (Ritalin) are also available. Methylxanthines include theophylline and caffeine, which are legal, but a variety of illegal stimulants is available. These drugs include amphetamines, which are synthetic (closely mimicking *Ephedra sinica*, the source of natural ephedrine), and cocaine, derived from coca leaves. A more recent addition to the illegal stimulant panacea includes cathinones, known as bath salts. Cathinones are the active ingredients in khat (*Catha edulis*), a leafy plant native to East Africa and the Arabian Peninsula.

Bath salts, mostly derivatives of cathinones, which had been synthesized in the 1920s, made a worldwide resurgence in the early 2000s. Mephedrone, methylenedioxypyrovalerone, and methylone are on Schedule I and illegal to possess in the

Table 1	
Effects observed with 25I-NBOMe	
Positive	Strong visuals, color shifts, euphoria, mental and physical energetic stimulation, increase in associative and creative thinking, increased awareness, life-changing spiritual experiences, feelings of love and empathy, body tingling sensation, increased sociability
Neutral	Pupil dilation, difficulty focusing, facial flushing, chills, goose bumps, change in perception of time, tachycardia, yawning, metallic chemical taste, sublingual numbness, hypertension, sweating
Negative	Agitation, confusion, scrambled communication, nausea, insomnia, paranoia, fear, panic, vasoconstriction, peripheral numbness, bodily shakes, grinding of teeth
Other	Rhabdomyolysis, deranged liver function

United States. However, new modifications of these substances are still widely prevalent.

Stimulants and cathinones have sympathomimetic effects. Signs and symptoms include sweating, palpitations, restlessness, tachycardia, nausea, chest pain, confusion, headache,[15] and, as reported later, psychosis. Skin changes (rash and bluish discoloration) can be seen, as well as changes in body odor.[16]

Stimulants are sought after because of desirable psychoactive effects such as increased energy, decreased appetite, and decreased sleep. They are as performance enhancers can be construed as an improvement in quality of life measures, for example, drinking caffeine or chewing khat leaves or coca leaves or being used as cognitive enhancers for academic performance. Some use, however, may result in severe addiction or psychiatric sequelae (or both), especially paranoia, hallucinations, and persecutory delusions. The steps toward addiction seem to hinge on the dose used and route of administration; faster onset of action is linked to increased likelihood for addiction, as are higher doses.[17,18] Cathinones represent a step closer to 3,4-methylenedioxy-methamphetamine, in that serotonergic action mitigates the overwhelmingly dopaminergic action of amphetamines and leads to a different quality high.

Stimulant use is higher in prevalence among individuals with psychosis, although it has been reported that lower amounts/frequency of use are sufficient to trigger psychosis in predisposed individuals. Despite variation in reported rates of psychosis in stimulant users, a pooled meta-analysis found that "Rates of stimulant use disorder were stable over time, and unrelated to age, sex, stage of psychosis, type of stimulant drug or study methodology factors."[19]

The mechanism of action of stimulants centers on catecholamines. Much interest has been focused on getting optimal performance enhancement without adverse effects given the extensive therapeutic use of this class. An activation continuum balances enhancement with minimization of adverse effects, following a U-shaped inverse curve.[20] Administration of high-dose stimulant results in decreased cognitive flexibility. Most stimulants are used for attention-deficit hyperactivity disorder. Bupropion, a well-known antidepressant also used for smoking cessation, is a weak cathinone-like derivative (**Fig. 3**).

Cocaine blocks the reuptake of monoamine neurotransmitters, including dopamine (DA), NE, and serotonin (5-HT). Blockade of DA reuptake is instrumental in the reinforcing and addictive properties of cocaine.[21] Amphetamine enters the cell through various monoamine reuptake transporters, reversing the vesicular monoamine transporter; this leads to a large release of cytoplasmic and vesicular stores of DA, NE, and 5-HT.[22] Synthetic cathinones, such as mephedrone and methylone, share a mechanism of action similar to amphetamines via monoamine reuptake inhibition, with some minor differences.[23] Thus, behavioral disturbances seen with stimulants are seen with cathinone derivatives as well (**Fig. 4**).[24]

SYNTHETIC CANNABINOIDS

Synthetic cannabinoids are a heterogeneous group of compounds that were first synthesized to study endogenous cannabinoid receptors but have since become popular drugs of abuse. In the 1960s, these substances were studied in an effort to separate the analgesic and anti-inflammatory properties of Δ9-tetrahydrocannabinol (Δ9-THC) from the psychotropic effects so that they could be used therapeutically. Professor John W. Huffman and his colleagues at Clemson University published some of the most comprehensive descriptions of these compounds beginning in the 1970s. More than 400 synthetic cannabinoids have since been developed, and many, such

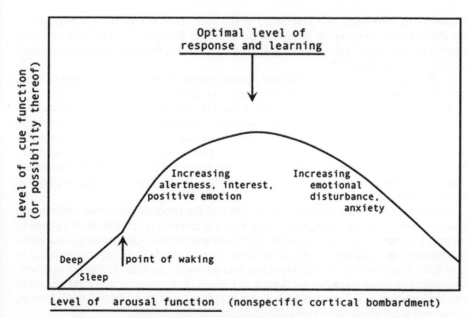

Fig. 3. Donald Hebb's optimal arousal theory, describing the continuum of activation of stimulants. Newer stimulants, for example, bath salts, cathinones, cause frequent behavioral disturbances consistent with Hebb's theory. (*From* Hebb DO. Drives and the C.N.S. (conceptual nervous system). Psychol Rev 1955;62:243–54. Image is in the public domain).

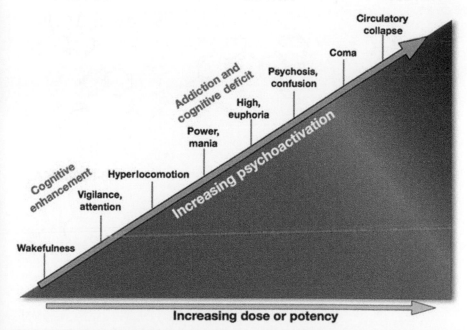

Fig. 4. Continuum of psychostimulant activation. (*From* Wood S, Sage JR, Shuman T, et al. Psychostimulants and cognition: a continuum of behavioral and cognitive activation. Pharmacol Rev 2014;66(1):195; with permission.)

as JWH-018, JWH-398, and JWH-412, reflect their origin in their names (**Fig. 5**).[25,26] By 2004, these compounds were being abused in Europe, and by 2008 they had spread to the United States, where they now rank among the most commonly abused psychoactive agents.[27–30]

Synthetic cannabinoids are typically sold as herbal mixtures in which one or more active drug has been dissolved in a solvent and applied to inert plant material.[31] In some circumstances, however, the plants used as the carrier have psychoactive effects of their own. The plant material is subsequently crushed and packaged for individual use. The product is most often smoked like marijuana, although it can also be taken orally. Several nicknames for these cannabinoid agonists exist, including Kush, Spice, K2, and legal weed. Oftentimes, specific blends of synthetic cannabinoids are sold under brand names, such as Black Mamba, White Tiger, Bonzai, and Master Kush[32,33] (**Fig. 6**).

Packaging generally contains a statement that the product contained within is not intended for human consumption and/or that the product is not intended for sale to minors. Merchants have attempted to use these warnings as protection against criminal prosecution. The legal status of synthetic cannabinoids is constantly evolving. In July 2012, the Controlled Substances Act was amended so that 15 different synthetic cannabinoids were classified as Schedule I drugs, indicating no currently accepted medical use and a high potential for abuse.[34] Subsequent laws passed at the federal, state, and local levels have criminalized additional compounds.[35,36]

Nevertheless, one reason synthetic cannabinoids are becoming increasingly popular is because users believe the products are legal weed. It also seems that some

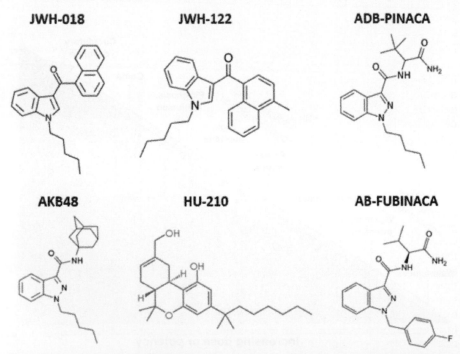

Fig. 5. Synthetic cannabinoid structure. (*From* Wiley JL, Marusich JA, Huffman JW. Moving around the molecule: relationship between chemical structure and in vivo activity of synthetic cannabinoids. Life Sci 2014;97:55–63.)

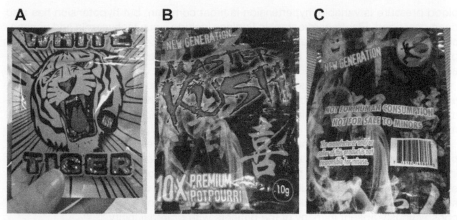

Fig. 6. (*A–C*) Examples of synthetic cannabinoids.

people are choosing synthetic cannabinoids over marijuana and other drugs of abuse because they wish to avoid detection from common urine drug screens. Other frequently cited explanations for synthetic cannabinoid use include attractive packaging, belief that these drugs are innocuous, and accessibility.[37]

It is inaccurate to refer to these psychoactive drugs as synthetic marijuana. Tetrahydrocannibinol, the primary psychoactive component of marijuana, is a partial agonist at cannabinoid CB_1 and CB_2 receptors. Agonism of CB_1 receptors produces alterations in mood, perception, and auditory and visual cognition. Agonism of CB_2 receptors, which are primarily located in immune tissue but which are also found in the central nervous system, stimulates immune cell motility and the release of immunomodulating substances. Synthetic cannabinoids seem to have even greater agonism at the CB_1 receptor than $\Delta9$-THC, which may explain the greater toxicity observed after abuse.[38] In addition, marijuana contains cannabidiol, which has been shown to mitigate the psychotomimetic effect of $\Delta9$-THC. Cannabidiol is not present in synthetic cannabinoids, which may explain the greater propensity toward psychosis.[39]

The tremendous heterogeneity of the compounds results in variable pharmacokinetic and pharmacodynamic effects. Indole- and pyrrole-derived synthetic cannabinoids have multiple sites where side chains can be added or substituted, and different combinations of constituents can produce significant differences in antinociceptive effect and locomotor activity.[40]

Psychiatric manifestations are the most consistent clinical findings in patients who present to the emergency department after synthetic cannabinoid abuse. Patients who achieve the desired sense of euphoria rarely require emergency treatment. Unfortunately, many patients have more significant reactions and may present with severe agitation reminiscent of stimulant abuse. Psychosis may manifest as paranoia, catatonia, illusions, or auditory or visual hallucinations.[41–44] Conversely, patients may present with decreased levels of unconsciousness and even unconsciousness. Other, more subtle neurologic abnormalities may be observed in synthetic cannabinoid toxicity, including tremor, nystagmus, fasciculations, and ataxia.[45] Generalized seizures have been attributed to synthetic cannabinoid abuse.[46–48] Cerebrovascular accident has also been reported.[49]

The most common cardiovascular manifestation of synthetic cannabinoid abuse is tachycardia, although patients may be normocardic or even bradycardic. Similarly, blood pressure is variable; hypertension is most common, but hypotension has also been described. Electrocardiographic findings include sinus tachycardia and nonspecific ST segment changes. Patients have presented with complaints of chest pain and palpitations, and myocardial infarction has been attributed to synthetic cannabinoid abuse.[50,51]

Other signs and symptoms of synthetic cannabinoid toxicity may include nausea and vomiting, pulmonary infiltrates, hypothermia or hyperthermia unrelated to environmental conditions, xerostomia, and pupil irregularities, including both mydriasis and miosis.[52–54]

There are no specific abnormalities of laboratory test results that typically accompany synthetic cannabinoid abuse, although there are many reports of acute kidney injury. The renal insufficiency may manifest as prerenal azotemia, acute tubular necrosis, or interstitial nephritis. Although many drug abusers are at risk for hypovolemia secondary to poor oral intake and/or significant diaphoresis, volume depletion is conspicuously absent in many of the patients with prerenal injury.[55–57]

Diagnosis is made by history and physical examination. The urine drug screens commonly used in most emergency departments do not test for synthetic cannabinoids, and these novel psychoactives do not produce a positive result on the readily available THC screen. There are new drug screens specifically designed to detect synthetic cannabinoids, but most emergency departments do not use them, and because new cannabinoids are constantly appearing, these tests quickly become obsolete. Comprehensive testing using liquid or gas chromatography in tandem with mass spectrometry can identify the exact xenobiotic, but this technology is not readily available in most health care settings.

EVALUATION AND MANAGEMENT IN THE EMERGENCY DEPARTMENT SETTING

The priority when assessing a patient under the influence of one of these novel psychoactives is ensuring the safety of the staff and other patients. Agitated patients may require isolation from the general population, sedation, and/or physical restraints.

Once safety is ensured, initial resuscitation consists of ensuring a patent airway and adequate breathing. Profound central nervous system depression can result in the loss of protective airway reflexes, and intubation should be performed if patients lack a gag reflex or cannot handle their secretions. Intubation is also advised for patients with hypercarbia or impaired oxygenation. Cervical spine precautions should be observed if there is any suspicion of trauma.

Hypertension and hypotension have both been observed in intoxicated patients. Hypertension requires emergent intervention only when there is evidence of end-organ damage. Adequate sedation is often sufficient to treat elevated blood pressure, but calcium channel antagonists and directly acting vasodilators have also been used successfully. Hypotension typically responds to boluses of intravenous crystalloid fluids. In refractory hypotension, the direct-acting NE is the preferred vasopressor. DA requires endogenous NE for its pressor effect, and many psychoactive medications inhibit the reuptake of serotonin, NE, and other catecholamines, rendering DA ineffective.

Reversible causes of altered mental status should be considered during the initial resuscitation. Blood glucose levels should be measured in anyone with abnormal mentation and in patients who have experienced a seizure. Naloxone administration should be considered in patients with central nervous system and respiratory depression. The use of flumazenil to reverse suspected benzodiazepine toxicity is controversial but may be helpful in cases of acute toxicity.[58]

Benzodiazepines are indicated for seizures having a toxicologic cause. Barbiturates are also effective, but phenytoin and levetiracetam are not recommended.

There are several approaches to sedating the acutely agitated patient. Although the combination of haloperidol, diphenhydramine, and lorazepam, colloquially referred to as a B-52, is commonly used, there are several disadvantages to this approach. Neither haloperidol nor lorazepam works rapidly when administered intramuscularly, which is the primary route of administration when intravenous access is lacking. One study found that the mean time to sedation for haloperidol was 28.3 minutes versus 32.2 minutes for lorazepam. Midazolam, conversely, had a mean time to sedation of 18.3 minutes.[59] In a similar study, sedation was achieved in 15 minutes using midazolam versus 30 minutes for both ziprasidone and droperidol.[60] Benzodiazepines have proved effective in the management of agitation whether the cause is substance abuse or withdrawal from ethanol or other γ-aminobutyric acid agonists and in psychosis. Antipsychotics successfully treat psychosis, but they have proved inferior in the management of withdrawal and are often ineffective in drug-induced agitation. For this reason, when the exact cause of the agitation is unknown, it may be more prudent to use rapid-acting benzodiazepines as monotherapy. Although droperidol has fallen out of favor, it has proved to be safe and more rapid acting.

Aggressive cooling is recommended for patients with hyperthermia. One safe, effective way to rapidly cool the patient is to disrobe the patient and place the patient on top of a cooling blanket. A wet sheet is then placed over the patient, and a large fan is placed at the bedside. Simultaneously using several methods of heat transmission can quickly lower body temperature to the desired temperature of 39°C.[61] Cooling to lower temperatures is not recommended because of the potential for inducing hypothermia and inducing shivering. Ice packs are also not advised because they can cause local tissue damage and stimulate systemic vasoconstriction.

Once the initial resuscitation has been completed, a more thorough assessment should occur. The history should elicit the substances, route, and dose used. Many of the newer drugs of abuse have street names that may be unfamiliar to the emergency physician. There are several online resources, including erowid.com, urbandictionary.com, and noslang.com/drugs/dictionary/, that may prove useful.

It is essential to take a thorough medical and psychiatric history because there may be similarities between substance abuse, primary psychiatric conditions, and medical conditions such as thyrotoxicosis and hepatic encephalopathy.

Physical examination should focus on vital signs and recognition of common toxidromes. Sympathomimetic toxicity, characterized by hypertension, tachycardia, mydriasis, agitation, diaphoresis, and hyperthermia, is observed in many patients abusing amphetamines and amphetamine-like compounds, such as synthetic cathinones. Serotonin toxicity often accompanies use of these substances and may present with tremor, clonus, hyperreflexia, shivering, confusion, and diaphoresis. Central nervous system depression, respiratory depression, and miosis are commonly exhibited by patients with opioid intoxication.

A careful inspection should be done for any injuries sustained while intoxicated or complications from drug abuse, including compartment syndrome and infections from intravenous use.

Laboratory tests may prove useful in the evaluation of a patient with altered mental status following drug use. Routine blood tests, such as the CBC, basic metabolic profile, liver profile, prothrombin time, and creatine phosphokinase level, may indicate end-organ complications from acute or chronic drug abuse. Thyroid studies may be considered in patients with unexplained tachycardia or bradycardia. Common ingestion laboratory tests, including ethanol, acetaminophen, and salicylates, are recommended if there is any indication of suicidal ideation.

Although screening for drugs of abuse is commonly performed on patients who present with altered mental status, its utility has been questioned.[62,63] False-positive results for amphetamine and methamphetamine have been attributed to labetalol, multiple antihistamines and phenothiazines, bupropion, and trazodone.[54,64,65] Cathinone derivatives may or may not produce a positive result. Dextromethorphan, venlafaxine, ibuprofen, and ketamine and its derivatives may produce false-positive results for phenycyclidine.[66–68] Few emergency departments screen for synthetic cannabinoids, and these compounds do not yield a positive result on the THC immunoassay. Comprehensive urine testing using thin-layer chromatography, liquid or gas chromatography, and mass spectroscopy can identify many of these xenobiotics, but few hospitals can perform this test emergently.

An electrocardiogram should be obtained on patients who are under the influence of drugs of abuse, and patients should remain on telemetry while symptomatic. Stimulants may produce dysrhythmia and infarction, and the presence of QT prolongation or QRS widening may influence decisions on pharmacotherapy.

Radiographic studies are rarely needed for patients who present with altered mental status following drug abuse. Computed tomographic scans of the head should be reserved for the following types of patients: (1) patients with known or suspected trauma, (2) patients with unexplained focal deficits, and (3) patients at high risk for intracranial catastrophes, such as people administered anticoagulation or antiplatelet therapy.

Chest radiography is also generally unnecessary and should be limited to patients with cardiopulmonary signs or symptoms and those with trauma to the chest.

There are several conditions that are often observed in patients who present under the influence of these novel psychoactive drugs. Rhabdomyolysis can result from prolonged immobilization or excessive psychomotor agitation. Intravenous fluid resuscitation is the initial treatment, but surgical consultation is recommended when there is concern for compartment syndrome. Acute kidney injury is often the result of volume depletion, but it may also be due to a direct nephrotoxic effect. Serotonin toxicity, characterized by spontaneous and inducible clonus, hyperreflexia, shivering, tremor, diaphoresis, hypertonicity, and altered mental status, is best treated with supportive care, including the use of benzodiazepines.[69] Patients in whom the condition is refractory may require the serotonin antagonist cyproheptadine, but this must be administered enterally by mouth or gastric tube.

Metabolic acidosis is treated with aggressive fluid resuscitation. Lactated Ringer solution is preferred over normal saline because large volumes of the latter can produce a hyperchloremic acidosis.[70–77]

EVALUATION AND MANAGEMENT IN THE OUTPATIENT SETTING

Once a patient is treated for intoxication, abuse, or withdrawal from substances in the emergency department, a provider must consider the next level of care. According to the psychiatric Diagnostic and Statistical Manual of Mental Disorders, Fifth Edition, a patient meets criteria for a substance use disorder if at least 2 or more of the following are present during a 12-month period:

- The substance is often taken in larger amounts or for a longer period than was intended.
- There is persistent desire or unsuccessful efforts to cut down or control substance use.

- A great deal of time is spent in activities necessary to obtain, use, or recover from the substance.
- There is craving or a strong desire or urge to use the substance.
- There is recurrent substance use resulting in a failure to fulfill major role obligations at work, school, or home.
- There is continued substance use despite having persistent or recurrent social or interpersonal problems caused or exacerbated by the substance use.
- Important social, occupational, or recreational activities are given up or reduced because of substance use.
- There is recurrent substance use in situations in which it is physically hazardous.
- Substance use is continued despite knowledge of having a persistent or recurrent physical or psychological problem that is likely to have been caused or exacerbated by the substance.
- There is tolerance, as defined by either of the following:
  o A need for markedly increased amounts of the substance to achieve intoxication or desired effect
  o A markedly diminished effect with continued use of the same amount of the substance
- There is withdrawal, as manifested by either of the following:
  o The characteristic withdrawal syndrome for the substance
  o The substance is taken to relieve or avoid withdrawal symptoms[78]

One major challenge may be the physician's awareness of a substance use disorder, whereas the patient may minimize or deny the problem. Public health approaches, such as Screening, Brief Intervention, and Referral to Treatment (SBIRT), may be helpful in identifying individuals who are at risk of developing (or have already developed) a substance use disorder. After screening, which may include use of questionnaires, if a patient is identified to be an at-risk individual, a brief intervention may follow, which could include techniques such as brief advice or use of motivational interviewing to help a patient understand how he or she is at risk. The severity of the substance use disorder may then influence the recommended follow-up options.[79] Although studies on the outcomes on alcohol use seem promising, the effect on illicit drug use is less studied; further studies are needed to determine any consistent benefits of SBIRT in illicit drug use.[80,81]

Other patients may already be cognizant of an existing substance use disorder or may already possess a strong desire to resume specialized treatment following relapse. Empathically reframing with a patient that relapse could be considered as a learning experience (as opposed to be a failure) may help to reduce patient shame. Understanding that addictions have a large inheritable predisposition, much like other medical diseases such as hypertension or diabetes, may help a provider empathize with a patient's condition. In fact, twin studies suggest that heritability of addictions ranges from 0.39 to 0.72.[82]

Options for treatment referrals may range from residential treatment to specialized outpatient options that include work with a therapist and/or mental health professional. Those with the highest risk of relapse may best be suited for residential treatment, if they are willing. Others may better fit with outpatient substance abuse treatment.

Oftentimes, those who use substances may have other mental disorders such as depression, anxiety, or bipolar or psychotic disorders.[83] These clients with co-occurring disorders often benefit most from treatment of both substance use disorders in addition to the underlying primary psychiatric disorders that may influence the use of substances. Referral to a psychiatrist may be a good option for those with co-occurring disorders.

Within outpatient treatment, one must consider both pharmacologic and counseling options. Various options for therapies that may be helpful regardless of the substance class type include self-help groups. One of the best known and utilized self-help groups are 12-step groups. These groups are commonly run under the names of Alcoholics Anonymous or Narcotics Anonymous and are self-run groups (without professionals) that follow the 12 steps, a blueprint on how to obtain sobriety. Twelve-step groups are spiritually based and focus on a higher power to help one to manage addiction. The benefits of 12-step groups are that they are ubiquitous, can be attended on a daily basis if desired, and do not require fee for attendance. They may provide an excellent support group and sober network. Although studies are heterogeneous about the use of 12-step groups and outcomes, they suggest the benefits of the groups.[84] Furthermore, meeting attendance and having a sponsor may correlate to abstinence in those who attend.[85]

Motivational interviewing is another therapeutic modality that may reduce substance use, compared with no intervention.[86] Motivational interviewing is an approach that assumes that direct confrontation of a patient's condition only leads to further resistance and denial. By taking a more client-centered approach that is nonjudgmental and exploratory, a provider may better help improve a patient's insight and increase the chance that a patient makes changes to the substance use. It is also crucial to understand that not everybody is motivated to change the using patterns and that people may be in different stages of motivation to change at any given time. Stages of motivation include the following:

1. Precontemplation: patient is in denial or does not believe that a problem exists.
2. Contemplation: patient is ambivalent about making a change about substance use. For example, the patient may state "yes I want to quit, but..."
3. Preparation: patient desires to make a change and is in the process of planning how to make the change.
4. Action: patient is actively making the change and may use the skills/resources provided.
5. Maintenance: patient has made the change and is working on prolonging the duration of changes.
6. Relapse: patient has gone back to using.

A provider may, through collaboration with the patient, guide the patient through these different stages until they reach maintenance. Although relapses may occur, it is important to understand that this is a natural part of the progression through treatment; the clinician can troubleshoot with the patient to take this as a learning experience. Similarly, if a patient remains in the precontemplative or contemplative stage, a provider may work toward building a patient's insight into the substance use disorder. It is expected that a patient's stage may fluctuate in time based on a patient's internal emotional state as well as external social factors.

Cognitive behavioral therapy and relapse prevention are other modalities that could help improve patient insights into identifying common high-risk triggers for substance use and how to avoid or live with them. Identifying maladaptive or distorted thought patterns or assumptions and learning to self-evaluate and adjust them is another aim of these therapies. Any of these therapy modalities may be done individually or in a group setting.

Unfortunately, at this time, for the substances mentioned in this article, there are no US Food and Drug Administration (FDA)-approved medications to help prolong sobriety or reduce heavy days of use. For treatment of amphetamine use disorders, some dopaminergic options such as bupropion and modafinil have shown some promise; however, there may not be enough supportive evidence at this time to recommend routine use.[87] There has also been some recent interest in the use of varenicline (a medication often used for smoking cessation) and its possible ability to attenuate the positive subjective effects of amphetamine.[88] However, future studies are needed to replicate these findings. It is also unknown if synthetic cathinone use disorders would respond to similar treatments, despite having amphetamine-like properties. For cannabis use disorders, there are no FDA-approved medications for treatment. Buspirone, lithium, divalproex, atomoxetine, and bupropion are among a few of the medications that have been studied. Buspirone has shown some promise in achieving a greater percentage of cannabis-negative urine samples, but this was from a smaller trial that would benefit from replication.[89] Although synthetic cannabinoids share the same actions with marijuana on CB_1 receptors, it is unknown if they would respond to the same treatments for cannabis use disorders.

It is important to monitor for signs of withdrawal or intoxication in the office. Although amphetamine-related withdrawal is not fatal, it can lead to symptoms such as anergia, increased appetite, or depressed mood. One must also be aware that sometimes amphetamine withdrawal leading to such dysphoric mood may warrant inpatient evaluation if significant suicidality occurs. Withdrawal does not typically occur from hallucinogens, NBOMe, or designer drugs. Although the existence of withdrawal from cannabis has been controversial in the past, it is now being recognized as a true clinical diagnosis. It may include anxiety, irritability, insomnia, restlessness, decreased appetite, and depressed mood. If a patient has acute medical symptoms, such as autonomic instability or seizures related to substance use, it would be most prudent to refer the patient to the emergency department for further management.

REFERENCES

1. Bersani FS, Corazza O, Albano G, et al. 25C-NBOMe: preliminary data on pharmacology, psychoactive effects, and toxicity of a new potent and dangerous hallucinogenic drug. Biomed Res Int 2014;2014:1–6.
2. Ninnemann A, Stuart GL. The NBOMe series: a novel, dangerous group of hallucinogenic drugs. J Stud Alcohol Drugs 2014;74(6):977–8.
3. Forrester M. NBOMe designer drug exposures reported to Texas poison centers. J Addict Dis 2014;33(3):196–201.
4. Case series: 7 patients with confirmed exposure to hallucinogenic stimulant 25I-NBOMe ("N-Bomb"). The Poison Review RSS Web site. 2013. Available at: http://www.thepoisonreview.com/2013/07/20/case-series-7-patients-with-confirmed-exposure-to-hallucinogenic-stimulant-25i-nbome-n-bomb/. Accessed March 26, 2015.
5. EMCDDA. Report on the risk assessment of 2-(4-iodo-2,5-dimethoxyphenyl)-N-(2-methoxybenzyl) ethanamine (25I-NBOMe) in the Framework of the Council Decision on New Psychoactive Substances. EMCDDA Web site. 2014. Available at: http://www.emcdda.europa.eu/publications/risk-assessment/25I-NBOMe. Accessed March 26, 2015.
6. Egan C, Herrick-Davis K, Miller K, et al. Agonist activity of LSD and lisuride at cloned 5HT 2A and 5HT 2C receptors. Psychopharmacology 1998;136(4):409–14.
7. Aghajanian G, Marek G. Serotonin and hallucinogens. Neuropsychopharmacology 1999;21(2S):S16–23.

8. Hanks J, González-Maeso J. Animal models of serotonergic psychedelics. ACS Chem Neurosci 2013;4(1):33–42.
9. Halberstadt A, Geyer M. Effects of the hallucinogen 2,5-dimethoxy-4-iodophene-thylamine (2C-I) and superpotent N-benzyl derivatives on the head twitch response. Neuropharmacology 2014;77:200–7.
10. Suzuki J, Poklis JL, Poklis A. "My friend said it was good LSD": a suicide attempt following analytically confirmed 25I-NBOMe ingestion. J Psychoactive Drugs 2014;46(5):379–82.
11. Grautoffand S, Kahler J. Near fatal intoxication with the novel psychoactive substance 25C-NBOMe. Med Klin Intensivmed Notfmed 2015;109(4):271–5.
12. Tang MH, Ching CK, Tsui MS, et al. Two cases of severe intoxication associated with analytically confirmed use of the novel psychoactive substances 25B-NBOMe and 25C-NBOMe. Clin Toxicol 2014;52(5):561–5.
13. Rose S, Poklis J, Poklis A. A case of 25I-NBOMe (25-I) intoxication: a new potent 5-HT2A agonist designer drug. Clin Toxicol 2013;51(3):174–7.
14. Zuba D, Sekuła K, Buczek A. 25C-NBOMe – new potent hallucinogenic substance identified on the drug market. Forensic Sci Int 2013;227(1–3):7–14.
15. Smith CD, Robert S. 'Designer drugs': update on the management of novel psychoactive substance misuse in the acute care setting. Clin Med 2014;14(4):409–15.
16. Wood D, Greene S, Dargan P. Clinical pattern of toxicity associated with the novel synthetic cathinone mephedrone. Emerg Med J 2011;28(4):280–2.
17. Koob GF, Volkow ND. Neurocircuitry of addiction. Neuropsychopharmacology 2010;35(1):217–38.
18. Dybdal-Hargreaves NF, Holder ND, Ottoson PE, et al. Mephedrone: public health risk, mechanisms of action, and behavioral effects. Eur J Pharmacol 2013;714(1–3):32–40.
19. Sara GE, Large M, Burgess P, et al. Stimulant use disorders in people with psychosis: a meta-analysis of rate and factors affecting variation. Aust N Z J Psychiatry 2014;49(2):106–17.
20. Hebb DO. Drives and the C.N.S. (conceptual nervous system). Psychol Rev 1955;62:243–54.
21. Goodman L. Drug addiction and drug abuse. In: Goodman & Gilman's the pharmacological basis of therapeutics. 11th edition. New York: McGraw-Hill; 2006.
22. Robertson S, Matthies H, Galli A. A closer look at amphetamine-induced reverse transport and trafficking of the dopamine and norepinephrine transporters. Mol Neurobiol 2009;39(2):73–80.
23. Nagai F, Nonaka R, Kamimura K. The effects of non-medically used psychoactive drugs on monoamine neurotransmission in rat brain. Eur J Pharmacol 2007;559(2–3):132–7.
24. Wood S, Sage JR, Shuman T, et al. Psychostimulants and cognition: a continuum of behavioral and cognitive activation. Pharmacol Rev 2014;66(1):193–221.
25. Thakur G, Nikas S, Makriyannis A. CB$_1$ cannabinoid receptor ligands. Mini Rev Med Chem 2005;5(7):631–40.
26. Matsuda L, Lolait S, Brownstein M, et al. Structure of a cannabinoid receptor and functional expression of the cloned cDNA. Nature 1990;279(Pt 1):561–4.
27. Forrester M, Kleinschmidt K, Schwarz E, et al. Synthetic cannabinoid and marijuana exposures reported to poison centers. Hum Exp Toxicol 2012;31(10):1006–11.
28. Bronstein A, Spyker D, Cantilena L, et al. Annual Report of the American Association of Poison Control Centers' National Poison Data System (NPDS): 25th Annual Report. Clin Toxicol 2008;46(10):927–1057.

29. Elliott S, Evans J. A 3-year review of new psychoactive substances in casework. Forensic Sci Int 2014;243:55–60.
30. Winstock A, Barratt M. Synthetic cannabis: a comparison of patterns of use and effect profile with natural cannabis in a large global sample. Drug Alcohol Depend 2013;131(1–2):106–11.
31. Zuba D, Byrska B, Maciow M. Comparison of "herbal highs" composition. Anal Bioanal Chem 2011;400:119–26.
32. Monte A, Bronstein A, Cao D, et al. An outbreak of exposure to a novel synthetic cannabinoid. N Engl J Med 2014;370:389–90.
33. Schifano F, Corazza O, Deluca P, et al. Psychoactive drug or mystical incense? Overview of the online available information on Spice products. Int J Cult Ment Health 2009;2:137–44.
34. United States Drug Enforcement Agency. USDEA Web site. Available at: http://www.deadiversion.usdoj.gov/21cfr/21usc/801.htm. Accessed March 20, 2015.
35. Federal Register. 2014. Available at: https://www.federalregister.gov/articles/2014/02/10/2014-02848/schedules-of-controlled-substances-temporary-placement-of-four-synthetic-cannabinoids-into-schedule. Accessed March 20, 2015.
36. Martin F. Houston City Council bans synthetic marijuana. Houston Public Media Web site. 2014. Available at: http://www.houstonpublicmedia.org/news/houston-city-council-bans-synthetic-marijuana-kush/. Accessed March 20, 2015.
37. Barratt M, Cakic V, Lenton S. Patterns of synthetic cannabinoid use in Australia. Drug Alcohol Rev 2013;32(2):141–6.
38. Fantegrossi WE, Moran JH, Radominska-Pandya A, et al. Distinct pharmacology and metabolism of K2 synthetic cannabinoids compared to D(9)-THC: mechanism underlying greater toxicity? Life Sci 2013;97:45–54.
39. Elsohly MA, Slade D. Chemical constituents of marijuana: the complex mixture of natural cannabinoids. Life Sci 2005;78:539–48.
40. Wiley JL, Marusich JA, Huffman JW. Moving around the molecule: relationship between chemical structure and in vivo activity of synthetic cannabinoids. Life Sci 2014;97:55–63.
41. Van der Veer N, Fiday J. Persistent psychosis following the use of Spice. Schizophr Res 2011;130(1–3):285–6.
42. Tung CK, Chiang TP, Lam M. Acute mental disturbance caused by synthetic cannabinoid: a potential emerging substance of abuse in Hong Kong. East Asian Arch Psychiatry 2012;22(1):31–3.
43. Hurst D, Loeffler G, McLay R. Psychosis associated with synthetic cannabinoid agonists: a case series. Am J Psychiatry 2011;168:1119.
44. Müller H, Huttner HB, Köhrmann M, et al. Panic attack after spice abuse in a patient with ADHD. Pharmacopsychiatry 2010;43:152–3.
45. Cohen J, Morrison S, Greenberg J, et al. Clinical presentation of intoxication due to synthetic cannabinoids. Pediatrics 2010;129:e1064–7.
46. Schneir AB, Cullen J, Ly BT. "Spice" girls: synthetic cannabinoid intoxication. J Emerg Med 2011;40:296–9.
47. Wells DL, Ott CA. The "new" marijuana. Ann Pharmacother 2010;45(3):414–7.
48. Lapoint J, James LP, Moran CL, et al. Severe toxicity following synthetic cannabinoid ingestion. Clin Toxicol (Phila) 2011;49:760–4.
49. Freeman MJ, Rose DZ, Myers MA, et al. Ischemic stroke after use of the synthetic marijuana "spice". Neurology 2013;81:2090–3.
50. Bebarta VS, Ramirez S, Varney SM. Spice: a new "legal" herbal mixture abused by young active duty military personnel. Subst Abus 2012;33:191–4.

51. Hoyte CO, Jacob J, Monte AA, et al. A characterization of synthetic cannabinoid exposures reported to the National Poison Data System in 2010. Ann Emerg Med 2012;60:435–8.
52. Canning JC, Ruha AM, Pierce R, et al. Severe GI distress after smoking JWH018. Clin Toxicol 2010;48:618.
53. Alhadi S, Tiwari A, Vohra R, et al. High times, low sats: diffuse pulmonary infiltrates associated with chronic synthetic cannabinoid use. J Med Toxicol 2013; 9:199–206.
54. Simmons JR. Intoxication from smoking "spice". Ann Emerg Med 2011;57(2): 187–8.
55. Bhanushali GK, Jain G, Fatima H, et al. AKI associated with synthetic cannabinoids: a case series. Clin J Am Soc Nephrol 2012;8:523–6.
56. Luciano RL, Perazella MA. Nephrotoxic effects of designer drugs: synthetic is not better! Nat Rev Nephrol 2014;10:314–24.
57. Centers for Disease Control and Prevention (CDC). Acute kidney injury associated with synthetic cannabinoid use–multiple states, 2012. MMWR Morb Mortal Wkly Rep 2013;62:93.
58. Seger DL. Flumazenil – treatment or toxin. J Toxicol Clin Toxicol 2004;42(2):209–16.
59. Nobay F, Simon BC, Levitt MA, et al. A prospective, double-blind, randomized trial of midazolam versus haloperidol versus lorazepam in the chemical restraint of violent and severely agitated patients. Acad Emerg Med 2004;11:744–9.
60. Martel M, Sterzinger A, Miner J, et al. Management of acute undifferentiated agitation in the emergency department: a randomized double-blind trial of droperidol, ziprasidone, and midazolam. Acad Emerg Med 2005;12:1167–72.
61. Wyndham CH, Strydom NB, Cooke HM, et al. Methods of cooling subjects with hyperpyrexia. J Appl Physiol 1959;14:771–6.
62. Tenenbein M. Do you really need that emergency drug screen? Clin Toxicol 2009; 47:286–91.
63. Wu AH, McKay C, Broussard LA, et al. National Academy of Clinical Biochemistry Laboratory Medicine Practice Guidelines: recommendations for the use of laboratory tests to support poisoned patients who present to the emergency department. Clin Chem 2003;49:357–79.
64. Yee LM, Wu D. False-positive amphetamine toxicology screen results in three pregnant women using labetalol. Obstet Gynecol 2011;117:503–6.
65. Huang BC, Lien MH, Wang PY, et al. Interference by drugs contained in over-the-counter cold syrups on methamphetamine immunoassay test kits used in drug abuse assessment. J Food Drug Anal 1995;34:259–68.
66. Budai B, Iskandar H. Dextromethorphan can produce false positive phencyclidine testing with HPLC. Am J Emerg Med 2002;20:61–2.
67. Schier J. Avoid unfavorable consequences: dextromethorphan can bring about a false-positive phencyclidine urine drug screen. J Emerg Med 2000;18:379–81.
68. Bond GR, Steele PE, Uges DR. Massive venlafaxine overdose resulted in a false positive Abbott AxSYM urine immunoassay for phencyclidine. J Toxicol Clin Toxicol 2003;41:999–1002.
69. Boyer EW, Shannon M. The serotonin syndrome. N Engl J Med 2005;352: 1112–20.
70. Skellet A, Mayer A, Durward A, et al. Chasing the base deficit: hyperchloraemic acidosis following 0.9% saline fluid resuscitation. Arch Dis Child 2000;83:514–6.
71. Scheingraber S, Rehm M, Sehmisch C, et al. Rapid saline infusion produces hyperchloremic acidosis in patients undergoing gynecologic surgery. Anesthesiology 1999;90:1265–70.

72. Kelly KL. Ranitidine cross-reactivity in the EMIT d.a.u. monoclonal amphetamine/methamphetamine assay. Clin Chem 1990;36:1391–2.
73. Melanson SE, Lee-Lewandrowski E, Griggs DA, et al. Reduced interference by phenothiazines in amphetamine drug of abuse immunoassays. Arch Pathol Lab Med 2006;130:1834–8.
74. Weintraub D, Linder MW. Amphetamine positive toxicology screen secondary to bupropion. Depress Anxiety 2000;12:53–4.
75. Olsen KM, Gulliksen M, Christophersen AS. Metabolites of chlorpromazine and brompheniramine may cause false positive urine amphetamine results with monoclonal EMIT d.a.u. immunoassay. Clin Chem 1992;38:611–2.
76. Kaim SC, Klett CJ, Rothfeld B. Treatment of the acute alcohol withdrawal state: a comparison of four drugs. Am J Psychiatry 1969;125:16406.
77. Amato L, Minozzi S, Vecchi S, et al. Benzodiazepines for alcohol withdrawal. Cochrane Database Syst Rev 2010;(3):CD005063.
78. American Psychiatric Association. Diagnostic and statistical manual of mental disorders. 5th edition. Arlington (VA): American Psychiatric Association; 2013.
79. Agerwala SA, McCance-Katz EF. Integrating screening, brief intervention, and referral to treatment (SBIRT) into clinical practice settings: a brief review. J Psychoactive Drugs 2012;44(4):307–17.
80. Madras BK, Compton WM, Avula D, et al. Screening, brief interventions, referral to treatment (SBIRT) for illicit drug and alcohol use at multiple healthcare sites: comparison at intake and six months. Drug Alcohol Depend 2009;99(1–3):280–95.
81. Woodruff SI, Clapp JD, Eisenberg K, et al. Randomized clinical trial of the effects of screening and brief intervention for illicit drug use: the Life Shift/Shift Gears study. Addict Sci Clin Pract 2014;9(1):8.
82. Ducci F, Goldman D. The genetic basis of addictive disorders. Psychiatr Clin North Am 2012;35(2):495–519.
83. Pettinati HM, O'Brien CP, Dundon WD. Current status of co-occurring mood and substance use disorders: a new therapeutic target. Am J Psychiatry 2013;170(1):23–30.
84. Kelly JF, Stout RL, Slaymaker V. Emerging adults' treatment outcomes in relation to 12-step mutual-help attendance and active involvement. Drug Alcohol Depend 2013;129(1–2):151–7.
85. Subbaraman ZM, Tonigan JS. Involvement in 12-step activities and treatment outcomes. Subst Abus 2013;34(10):60–9.
86. Smedslund G, Berg RC, Hammerstrom KT, et al. Motivational interviewing for substance abuse. Cochrane Database Syst Rev 2011;(5):CD008063.
87. Brensilver M, Heinzerling KG, Shoptaw S. Pharmacotherapy of amphetamine-type stimulant dependence: an update. Drug Alcohol Rev 2013;32(5):449–60.
88. Verrico CD, Mahoney JJ, Thompson-Lake DG, et al. Safety and efficacy of varenicline to reduce positive subjective effects produced by methamphetamine in methamphetamine-dependent volunteers. Int J Neuropsychopharmacol 2014;17(2):223–33.
89. Weinstein AM, Gorelick DA. Pharmacological treatment of cannabis dependence. Curr Pharm Des 2011;17(14):1351–8.

Shift, Interrupted: Strategies for Managing Difficult Patients Including Those with Personality Disorders and Somatic Symptoms in the Emergency Department

Nidal Moukaddam, MD, PhD[a,*], Erin AufderHeide, MD[b],
Araceli Flores, PhD[a], Veronica Tucci, MD, JD[b]

KEYWORDS

- Difficult patients • Somatic symptoms • Personality • Bias • Countertransference

KEY POINTS

- Difficult patients are often those who present with a mix of psychiatric and physical issues, such as somatoform disorders, and seem refractory to treatment and/or reassurance. Psychological factors can exacerbate physical complaints.
- Patients with personality disorders, especially cluster B personality disorder (borderline, histrionic, antisocial), can be manipulative and drug seeking or have repeated self-harm attempts.
- Patients with cluster A personality disorder can be frankly paranoid and need to be screened for psychosis.
- A difficult patient encounter can also be due to provider feelings, bias, or countertransference (CT). If a provider feels negatively about a patient, workup may be substandard, and dangerous medical mistakes can be made.

INTRODUCTION

Lisa: *"You know, there's too many buttons in the world. There's too many buttons and they're just - There's way too many just begging to be pressed, they're just begging to be pressed, you know? They're just - they're just begging to be pressed, and it makes*

Disclosure Statement: The authors have nothing to disclose.
[a] Menninger Department of Psychiatry and Behavioral Sciences, Baylor College of Medicine, 1502 Taub Loop, NPC Building 2nd Floor, Houston, TX 77030, USA; [b] Section of Emergency Medicine, Baylor College of Medicine, 1504 Taub Loop, Houston, TX 77030, USA
* Corresponding author.
E-mail address: nidalm@bcm.edu

me wonder, it really makes me…wonder, why doesn't anyone ever press mine? Why am I so neglected? Why doesn't anyone reach in and rip out the truth and tell me that I'm a…whore, or that my parents wish I were dead?"

Susanna: *"Because you're dead already, Lisa! No one cares if you die, Lisa, because you're dead already. Your heart is cold. That's why you keep coming back here. You're not free. You need this place, you need it to feel alive. It's pathetic. I've wasted a year of my life. Maybe everybody out there is a liar. And maybe the whole world is 'stupid' and 'ignorant'. But I'd rather be in it…than down here with you."*[1]

In the 1999 feature film Girl, Interrupted, Winona Rider and Angelina Jolie offered gut-wrenching portrayals of Susanna Kaysen and Lisa Rowe, respectively. Susanna was an 18-year-old patient admitted to an inpatient psychiatric ward and diagnosed with borderline personality disorder after a haphazard suicide attempt. Lisa, another patient in the ward, is described as a charming, manipulative, and, ultimately, unstable woman who was diagnosed as a sociopath.

Both women in the film and Susanna Kaysen's 1993 autobiographical account epitomize difficult patients that Emergency personnel cringe when encountering. Indeed, after viewing the film, one emergency department (ED) nurse remarked, "Every time I encounter one of these girls, I feel another part of my soul die."

What Makes a Patient Difficult?

Clinical encounters represent the beginning, and the heart of, the treatment process. Despite remarkable advances in medicine and technology, the process starts with a simple clinical interview, which, in turn, determines subsequent medical decision making. As such, the clinical interview is the gateway for the remainder of medical care, and although most clinical interviews proceed unimpeded, there are certain groups of difficult patients whose care is challenging. This article reviews 3types of commonly encountered difficulties summarized in **Fig. 1**.

The first is somatic symptoms masquerading as psychiatric and/or seemingly untreatable symptoms. In this case, the difficulty is of diagnostic nature. The emergency medicine literature commonly refers to these as somatoform, although the psychiatric technical meaning of this term is different as outlined later.

Second, patient encounters can be difficult because of personality traits or disorders. In this case, the difficulty stems from the patient. Such patients can be entitled, demanding, demeaning, or clingy. They may be resistant to routine treatment, threaten self-harm, and display manipulative or drug-seeking behaviors.

Lastly, some clinical encounters are complicated by provider feelings. Bias on behalf of the provider, or burnout, which is unfortunately common in modern health care, can make patient encounters feel heavy and unpleasant. This area is complicated and

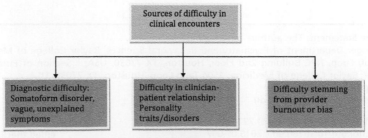

Fig. 1. Sources of difficulty in clinical encounters.

poorly understood but, as any clinician can attest, is crucial to being an effective, caring treatment provider.

Dealing with difficult patients is not a new challenge in medicine. As outlined by Groves in 1978,[2] at least 4 types of difficult patients exist: the dependent clinger, the entitled demander, the manipulative help rejecter, and the self-destructive denier, but this classification does not meet the demands of modern health care anymore, as outlined later.

In summary, somatic symptoms and personality disorders presenting to the ED can be particularly challenging for health care providers secondary to inadequate management, recurrent presentation for the same symptoms, and physician frustration with inability to provide a cure.

SOMATOFORM DISORDERS: DIAGNOSTIC DIFFICULTY AND POOR RESPONSE TO ROUTINE TREATMENTS

The cost of burden of psychiatric illness is substantial, with mental illness being the leading cause of disability-adjusted life years worldwide and accounting for 37% of healthy years lost from noncommunicable diseases.[3] This section introduces the definition of somatoform disorders and also includes common diagnostic pitfalls masquerading as somatoform issues.

Definitions and Alternate Terminology

The Emergency Medicine literature classically refers to physical symptoms presenting secondary to psychological distress as somatoform disorders.[4] Manifestations of psychological distress as a physical ailment is categorized as a distinct entity from malingering, in that the patient's symptoms are not intentionally feigned. The psychiatric literature used to classify somatoform disorders into somatization disorder, conversion disorder, hypochondriasis, pain disorder, body dysmorphic disorder, undifferentiated somatoform disorder, somatoform disorder not otherwise specified.

However, the traditional term somatoform disorders used in the Diagnostic and Statistical Manual of Mental Disorders (DSM)-III and DSM-IV has been changed to somatic symptoms and related disorders (new DSM-V terminology), with new additional diagnostic criteria.[5] The DSM-IV diagnosis of somatization disorder required a specific number of complaints from among 4 symptom groups. The DSM-V criteria do not have such a requirement; instead, the main requirement is that somatic symptoms must be "significantly distressing or disruptive to daily life and must be accompanied by excessive thoughts, feelings, or behaviors."

DSM-V has also introduced a new disorder, illness anxiety disorder, reminiscent of the older hypochondria term, the core symptom of which is worry about having an illness and not being easily placated by negative tests or verbal reassurance. According to the DSM-V, the previous set of criteria (DSM-IV) emphasized the unexplained nature of medical symptoms rather than the accompanying distress. The distinctions between the old criteria under the DSM-IV and the new criteria in the DSM-V are summarized on **Table 1**.

The term medically unexplained physical symptoms (MUPS) has also been used to describe somatic complaints mentioned earlier.[6] Patients may think that their symptoms (and underlying problems) are not appreciated or fully treated, and this may quickly lead to an antagonistic physician-patient relationship, repeated emergency room visits, and unhappy patients.

For the sake of simplicity, in this article, the term somatoform disorders is used as an umbrella term to describe somatic symptoms and related disorders.

Table 1
Comparison of DSM-IV somatoform disorders and DSM-V somatic symptoms and related disorders

DSM-IV: Categories of Somatoform Disorders	Criteria to Meet Diagnosis	DSM-V: Somatic Symptoms & Related Disorders	Criteria to Meet Diagnosis
Somatization disorder	• Symptoms manifest before age 30 y, symptoms last several years, and symptoms impair social or occupational function • One of the following in addition to the above-mentioned criteria during any time of the course of the disorder: 　1. Four pain symptoms 　2. Two pain symptoms 　3. One sexual symptom or 　4. One pseudoneurologic symptom	Somatic symptom disorder	• One or more somatic symptoms that are distressing or cause a disruption in daily life • Excessive thoughts, feelings, or behaviors related to the somatic symptom • Patient is symptomatic for more than 6 mo, even if physical symptom is not consistently present
Conversion disorder	Presentation of neurologic symptoms that cannot be explained by a medical condition (ie, paralysis, blindness, hearing loss, numbness)	Conversion disorder	• One or more symptoms of altered voluntary motor or sensory function • Clinical evidence incompatible between symptom and recognized medical conditions • The symptom or deficit not better explained by another disorder • Clinically significant distress or impairment in functioning

Hypochondriasis	Preoccupation with concern for a serious medical problem when no such condition exists	Illness anxiety disorder	• Preoccupation with acquiring a serious illness • Somatic symptoms not present or mild if present • High level of anxiety about health • Excessive health-related behaviors or maladaptive avoidance • Illness preoccupation for at least 6 mo • Illness-related preoccupation not better explained by another mental disorder
Pain disorder	Pain that causes significant stress or impairment in functioning	Psychological factors affecting other medical conditions	• A medical symptom or disorder is present • Psychological or behavioral factors affect the medical condition in one or several ways • The psychological and behavioral factors are not better explained by another mental disorder
Body dysmorphic disorder	Obsession with or exaggeration of minor or perceived flaws	Factitious disorder	• Falsification of symptoms or induction of injury associated with identified deception • The individual presents as ill or injured, impaired • Absence of external rewards • Behavior not better explained by another mental disorder
Undifferentiated somatoform disorder	• One or more symptom that causes significant distress or impairs functioning • Symptoms last at least 6 mo	Other specified somatic symptom and related disorder	This category includes brief versions of the above-mentioned criteria as well as pseudocyesis (false belief of being pregnant)
Somatoform disorder not otherwise specified	Somatic symptoms that do not meet any of the criteria specified for the other somatoform disorders	—	—

Adapted from American Psychiatric Association. Diagnostic and statistical manual of mental disorders. 5th edition. Washington, DC: American Psychiatric Publication; 2013; and American Psychiatric Association. Diagnostic and Statistical Manual of Mental Disorders. 4th ed. Washington, DC: American Psychiatric Association; 1994.

Emergency physicians (EPs) are tasked with sifting through a myriad of chief complaints to determine which arise from organic disorders, including those that pose an imminent threat to the patient's life, and which are psychosomatic in origin. Emergency providers are often limited in their ability to holistically address all the contributing factors in patients presenting with somatic complaints. However, an organized approach to thoroughly evaluate for organic causes of patient symptoms, while simultaneously avoiding potentially harmful and unwarranted diagnostic studies, can lead to improved patient care and increased satisfaction on the part of both the physician and patient. Caution must be taken that the physician does not jump to conclusions that the patient is faking or malingering. Medicine is fraught with unexplained symptoms that become well understood as knowledge advances. One glaring example is the discovery of *Helicobacter pylori*, before which so many individuals were diagnosed with stress ulcers.

Cultural factors can also play a role in the presentation of somatic symptoms. For example, complaining of pain such as gastrointestinal disturbance may be the only culturally acceptable way of seeking care for psychological disorders when the patient's true, underlying condition is depression. Somatic symptoms can serve as a gateway to the diagnosis of mood or other disorders, and on screening, multiple other socioeconomic issues may come to light as well.

The Mind-Body Connection: Which Symptoms Present to the Emergency Room?

A multitude of seemingly organic chief complaints can present to the emergency center (EC) veiled as somatizing (psychologically driven) symptoms, and conversely, conditions that appear psychiatric in nature can be a manifestation of a serious underlying organic disease.

Organic illnesses may also have complex presentations. Throughout history, vague and unusual symptoms were attributed to psychiatric conditions. Only with advances in science were these conditions discovered to be true organic pathologic conditions. Diseases that have the potential to be mistaken for a somatoform include endocrine disorders (ie, hyperthyroidism, thyroid disorders, Addison disease, insulinoma, panhypopituitarism), hereditary metabolic disorders (Wilson disease, urea cycle disorders, homocystinuria, creatine deficiency syndromes, Niemann-Pick disease type C, cerebrotendinous xanthomatosis), poisonings (ie, botulism, heavy metals, carbon monoxide), multiple sclerosis, systemic lupus erythematosus, and myasthenia gravis.[7–13] These madness mimickers are further summarized in **Table 2**.

As with most presenting symptoms to the ED, a complete and thorough history and physical examination (H&P) are paramount to adequately manage and treat the presenting symptoms. The following 3 sections addressing chest pain, abdominal pain, and blindness highlight how ED physicians might use clinical decision algorithms, H&P, and specific tests to evaluate for both organic and psychiatric pathology as the root cause of the patient's symptoms. Commonly seen symptoms in the ED that have the potential to mask psychological issues are also discussed.

Common Somatic Symptom: Chest Pain

Chest pain is a common somatic symptom but nevertheless could also represent a potentially life-threatening cause. In addition to careful H&P, vital signs, basic and specific laboratory tests, electrocardiogram, and clinical gestalt, clinical decision-making rules such as thrombolysis in myocardial infarction score, heart score, pulmonary embolism rule-out criteria, and Well criteria, for acute coronary syndromes and

Table 2
Madness mimickers

Psychiatric Symptoms/Common Psychiatric Misdiagnosis	Associated Symptoms	Hereditary Metabolic Disorder[1]
Behavioral abnormalities, impulsivity, mania, depression → bipolar or schizoaffective disorder, personality disorder, inebriation	Intermittent pain, particularly abdominal pain Patients can also present with tetraplegia (commonly misdiagnosed as Guillain-Barré syndrome)	Acute intermittent porphyria
Behavioral abnormalities, depression → bipolar disorder, depression	Extrapyramidal symptoms, dysarthria, akinesia	Wilson disease
Behavioral abnormalities, confusion, hallucinations → bipolar disorder	Headache, abdominal pain, changes in diet	Urea cycle disorders
Behavioral abnormalities, obsessive compulsive behavior, disinhibition → personality disorder	Ectopia lentis, marfanoid appearance, mental deficiency thrombosis	Homocysteinuria
Behavioral abnormalities, aggressiveness → personality disorder	Mental deficiency, language delay, epilepsy, extrapyramidal symptom	Creatine deficiency syndrome
Confusion, delusions → atypical psychosis	Ataxia, abnormal movements, supranuclear gaze palsy	Niemann-Pick disease type C
Delusions, hallucinations → schizophrenia	Juvenile cataract, tendinous xanthomata, cerebellar ataxia, spastic paraplegia, dementia	Cerebrotendinous xanthomatosis

pulmonary embolism, respectively, can assist emergency medicine in eliminating the need to undergo more invasive and unnecessary testing.

As chest pain is potentially a life-threatening symptom, it must be treated as such and psychiatric causes are a diagnosis of exclusion. Gastroesophageal reflux disease is the most common cause of noncardiac chest pain[11] and is often worked up on an outpatient basis.

Psychological comorbidity, including panic disorder anxiety and major depression, is also common, with a prevalence of up to 75% in patients presenting with noncardiac chest pain.[10,12] Psychiatric conditions can both mimic and exacerbate cardiac chest pain, and caution should be taken when attributing psychiatric conditions as the cause of chest pain.

Cognitive behavioral therapy (CBT) has been used to successfully treat panic disorders[14,15] and, therefore, may also be a consideration for patients with noncardiac chest pain. Several studies have shown that CBT is effective in treating noncardiac chest pain. An empirical treatment of antidepressants (venlafaxine, sertraline, and imipramine) can also be beneficial in patients with noncardiac chest pain.[16]

Only after a thorough workup with negative results should the EP entertain the notion that the patient's chest pain and shortness of breath are somatic manifestations of undiagnosed anxiety and depression. If such a determination is made, the EP should be mindful that effective therapy for anxiety and depression includes outpatient follow-up and treatment with antidepressants and antianxiety medications, or alternative therapies can be initiated in the ED in consultation with psychiatric providers.

Common Somatic Symptom: Abdominal Pain

Abdominal pain may also represent a potentially life-threatening cause, and in the geriatric population, abdominal pathology presenting to the ED carries a mortality approaching 10%.[17,18] Nevertheless, abdominal pain becomes a particularly mystifying and frustrating symptom, for both patient and physician, particularly when basic abdominal laboratory tests, lipase levels, liver function tests, bedside ultrasonography, and a thorough H&P fail to elucidate a cause. Irritable bowel syndrome (IBS) is thought to have some psychosomatic component, and a large number of patients with IBS have concurrently diagnosed anxiety, depression, or other mental health disorder. Screening for concurrent mental health disorders and referring patients to proper mental health treatment, when appropriate, can ameliorate somatic symptoms.[19]

Acute intermittent porphyria, traditionally called the royal malady because King George III is believed to have suffered from this disease, is another example of madness mimicker[19]: acute intermittent porphyria is autosomal dominant and caused by a deficiency in the enzyme porphobilinogen deaminase, which is involved in the biosynthesis of heme. Attacks of acute intermittent porphyria can be triggered by oral contraceptives, barbiturates, antiepileptics, sepsis, or alcohol.[2] Diagnosis is made by measurement of urine porphobilinogen levels, which are greatly increased during attacks but may be normal between attacks, and treatment involves both infusion of heme arginate and removal of any exogenous triggers (ie, oral contraceptive pills, barbiturates, antiepileptics, alcohol).[20]

Challenging Somatic Symptom: Blindness

Unlike chest pain and abdominal pain, sudden-onset blindness is not a complaint encountered on a daily basis in the ED, making it easier for the EP to ascertain whether it is a somatic finding or an "organic zebra" (ie unusual finding) such as an optic chiasm tumor. To make this determination, the EP can use the optokinetic reflex test, in which a black and white striped paper is flashed horizontally in front of the patient's face when the patient is asked to keep his or her eyes open and maintain a forward gaze. An individual with sight cannot help but track the paper and exhibits nystagmus.

Although psychological therapy and physical approaches seem to improve patients' symptoms,[21,22] there is no definitive consensus, even among experts, regarding the best treatment of patients with conversion disorder.[23]

Management and Diagnostic Considerations

The aforementioned chief complaints categorized as somatic complaints are diagnoses of exclusion. The EC physician who classifies a patient's symptoms as somatic without thorough investigation risks not only missing a true organic pathologic condition but also leads to potential future bias in equating any new symptoms to a purely psychosomatic cause. Nevertheless, the clinician who is able to assess for possible underlying psychosomatic components can greatly aid patients by both sparing them unnecessary future testing and unnecessary medical costs and simultaneously offering tools that appropriately address the patient's somatic symptoms.

Unfortunately, there is no consensus on the treatment of conversion disorder. However, many patients respond positively to explanation of symptoms as a manifestation of psychosocial stressors.[22] Resolution of symptoms on reassurance is not uncommon in a patient presenting with conversion disorder. As conversion disorder has an underlying psychosocial component, treatment based on combating comorbid psychiatric disorders and social stressors can also be effective. In addition, physical therapy (PT) has shown promising results of treatment of conversion disorder, and in some patients, complete resolution of symptoms following PT has been noted.[24,25]

The interview is the most effective strategy for diagnosis in somatization disorders, and again, the EC physician makes determination of what needs workup and not, so rare conditions have the potential to be missed. Consideration of other organic disorders that may present similarly to somatization is important.

PATIENTS WITH DIFFICULT PERSONALITIES

To complicate matters, patients presenting to the ED with somatic symptoms have a high prevalence of underlying personality disorders. Personality disorders are characterized by an enduring pattern of behavior (inflexible and pervasive), which deviates from cultural expectations and is manifest through a maladaptive pattern of perceiving and relating to others. It is estimated that up to 67% of patients with somatoform disorders have personality disorders as well, making this group particularly difficult to deal with.[26]

The personality clusters and subcategorizations are noted in **Table 3**. Each of the 3 personality clusters and subcategorized personality disorders may have distinct ways of manifesting their own psychological distresses as shown in **Fig. 2**. These patients' maladaptive patterns of perceiving and relating to others can serve as a barrier to receiving adequate evaluation for organic symptoms as well as promote exacerbation of somatic symptoms.

A label of personality disorder may contribute to a patient's complaint being dismissed without proper workup. Cluster A personality disorders may present with distrust, suspiciousness, paranoia, or eccentric beliefs. It is essential to rule out psychotic disorders when appropriate. Cluster B personality disorders, on the other hand, often have complicated trajectories within health care, as individuals with antisocial personality disorder may present with manipulative, drug-seeking behavior, those with borderline personality disorders may be seen repeatedly with self-harm attempts, and histrionic patients crave attention.

Not much is known about cluster C personality disorders in health care, as these individuals may not cause much provider distress. However, in individuals with obsessive-compulsive personality disorders, excessive perfectionism, rigidity, and stubbornness can easily complicate care by leading to decreased compliance and frequent questioning of medical decisions.

Despite the challenges inherent in dealing with difficult patients, the emergency medicine physician must adequately evaluate for an organic disorder while simultaneously avoiding bias by categorizing a psychiatric patient as someone who does not have the potential to suffer organic pathologic conditions. Bias in the medical profession is such that many patients with mental illness are more likely to have undiscovered organic pathologic conditions because their symptoms were attributed to psychiatric and not

Table 3		
Personality disorder clusters and subcategorizations		
Cluster A Personality Disorders	**Cluster B Personality Disorders**	**Cluster C Personality Disorders**
Paranoid	Borderline	Avoidant
Schizoid	Narcissistic	Dependent
Schizotypal	Histrionic	Obsessive-compulsive
	Antisocial	—

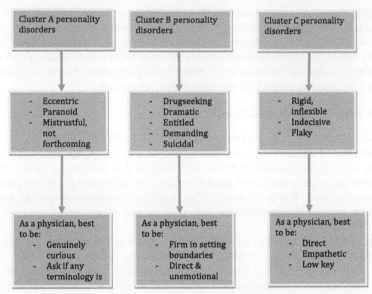

Fig. 2. Common presentations and strategies for personality disorders.

medical disease. Nevertheless, an expensive workup with computed tomography angiography or trip to the catheterization laboratory, for example, is not warranted nor advised on every single patient who presents to the ED with chest pain. Therefore, the EP walks a fine line between repeated evaluation of somatic symptoms for possible life-threatening causes and the determination that a particular patient's physical complaint does not warrant further medical investigation.

As a general rule, EPs cannot and should not prematurely diagnose a patient with a personality disorder from a single interview, as it often takes outpatient psychiatrists several visits to ascertain such a serious diagnosis. Even in the setting of return visits or so-called frequent fliers, the ED environment is inadequate for such diagnoses.

DIFFICULTY CAUSED BY PROVIDER FEELINGS—BIAS AND COUNTERTRANSFERENCE

Sometimes, the clinical interview is complicated because the provider is struggling with the case at hand. This situation could manifest as impatience, irritability, and inability to control one's emotions. In many cases, the patients encountered in emergency medicine practice are difficult. However, some clinical encounters are complicated by a provider's emotional temperature.

Medical decision making is not an objective process, despite the presence of medical algorithms for workup and diagnosis of most conditions. Bias in medical decision making can cause costly mistakes in treatment and has been linked to race, gender, and socioeconomic status. The real reasons for bias are not well understood nor are the mechanisms by which bias affects decision making. It is known, however, that physician state of mind, biases, and preconceived opinions can strongly shape any therapeutic encounter.

Countertransference

CT is a psychodynamic term dating back to Sigmund Freud, the founder of psychoanalysis. CT, the psychodynamic concept representing feelings of providers toward patients, has been reported anecdotally to affect decision making. Literature on hateful patients and hateful physicians is commonplace.[27] Modern CT representations have operationalized CT feelings into 8 dimensions: overwhelmed/disorganized, helpless/inadequate, positive, special/overinvolved, sexualized, disengaged, parental/protective, and criticized/mistreated.[28] Preliminary data (Moukaddam and Tucci, unpublished data, 2015) suggest that CT affects medical decision making in everyday patient encounters, not exclusively in psychiatric settings. The effect is most prominent when the criticized/mistreated, helpless/inadequate dimensions are activated. The effect is less pronounced when a diagnostic dilemma is absent, as in the case of the patient with a bone fracture or an open wound. When providers had positive CT for a patient, less testing for substance use or alcohol may be performed. Lack of awareness of one's own feelings toward patients could cause significant changes in treatment, potentially missing serious conditions.

Management Goals

Once the determination has been made that the patient's symptoms are not secondary to an organic pathologic condition, a more appropriate management strategy can be used.

General management strategies can help to ameliorate possible tension between physician and patient and provide patients with some relief regarding the cause of their symptoms. Sharing the diagnostic uncertainty, when appropriate, is also helpful. Explaining symptoms using socially acceptable terms (eg, muscle tension, stress, hyperventilation) rather than with a purely psychiatric explanation can also help the patient grapple with their own symptomatology. For example, certain serious heart conditions such as Takotsubo cardiomyopathy (or broken heart syndrome) do have an underlying psychological component. Therefore, discussing the link between physical and emotional health when addressing a possible somatic symptom can be reassuring to some patients in that it legitimizes their symptoms.

The goal of management of both somatizing symptoms and personality disorders, unlike other disorders presenting to the ED, focuses on providing not only a cure to the patients' ailments but also a sympathetic ear through active listening, validating the patients' concerns, and focusing on strategies for managing their symptoms and/or maladaptive patterns. Mindfulness is one such effective strategy that has been used to manage symptoms.[29]

Screening for underlying mental issues and consultation to psychiatry, when appropriate, can also help, as many patients with somatic symptoms have underlying psychiatric issues. These coexistent psychiatric disorders exacerbate somatic symptoms.

Setting realistic expectations for the alleviation of symptoms is paramount in that unrealistic expectations on the part of the patient manifests as disappointment, frustration, and discord in future physician-patient relationships. For most patients, total alleviation of symptoms is unrealistic, and for the patient with chronic somatization disorder, total alleviation of symptoms can, ironically, be met with hostility.

The exception is young patients with no underlying medical or psychiatric illness who present with symptoms as a result of a clear stressful life event. These patients respond well to reassurance and explanation of their symptoms, and channeling them into proper mental health care is essential.

Pharmacologic Strategies

Addictive pain medications such as narcotics and anxiolytics (eg, benzodiazepines) are contraindicated in patients whose symptoms are suspected to have a psychological/personality cause. If pain medications must be given, they should be nonaddictive medications and given on a scheduled basis rather than as needed. Gabapentin can be used for the treatment of anxiety and for the treatment of alcohol dependence.[30,31] Hydroxyzine, a first-generation antihistamine, has been used with success for the treatment of anxiety.[32] Pregabalin is frequently used for generalized anxiety disorder.[32,33] However, both gabapentin and pregabalin have a small, but meaningful, abuse potential.

If a mood disorder such as depression, or an anxiety disorder, is comorbid with somatoform or personality disorders, effectively treating the former can help significantly.

An empirical treatment of antidepressants should be considered in patients presenting with somatic symptoms of anxiety or depression, such as chest pain. Antidepressants and tricyclic antidepressants have been effective in the treatment of physical symptoms, anxiety, and depression without significant difference in efficacy between the 2 classes. Nevertheless, any medication comes with potential side effects, and the potential benefit versus potential harm with the implementation of any new medication regimen must be considered. Natural products such as St. John's wort have been shown to significantly reduce physical symptoms when compared with placebo.[16]

Starting use of psychotropic medications in the ED can be difficult in that these medications do not typically exhibit beneficial effects quickly and must be followed up by a primary psychiatric or primary care provider. If psychotropic medications are given in the ED, the patient should have a close follow-up to be able to assess the efficacy of the medications and make adjustments as needed.

Nonpharmacologic Strategies

A supportive health care provider is essential to the effective treatment of both somatoform and personality disorders. Many patients with somatization resist being referred to psychiatrist, as they feel that their concerns are being devalued. Consultation with a psychiatrist, nonetheless, is appropriate for confirmation of diagnosis as well as for the discussion of medications (for possible comorbid psychiatric conditions) that may help to alleviate somatoform symptoms.

Management is best carried out with a single provider, who is able to manage medications for possible concurrent psychiatric conditions as well as help patients with personality disorders better cope with maladaptive patterns.[4]

Psychotherapy, particularly CBT, is beneficial for patients with somatic symptoms and personality disorders, as well as MUPS. Therapy skills such as mindfulness-based exercises, emotional regulation, and distress tolerance can help patients better cope with symptoms. Although long-term therapy is not feasible in 1 visit, skills can be taught. Examples of CBT techniques are behavioral activation, problem solving, and relaxation training. Mindfulness techniques have also shown similar results in treatment of somatic symptoms.[33] In addition, meditation techniques have been shown to be beneficial for patients with somatization.[34,35] Thus, referrals to outpatient psychological services for individual/group therapy may also be an option if multidisciplinary collaboration is available.

Addressing specific symptoms and offering benign management strategies for those symptoms can provide some relief to patients (ie, treating back pain with a heating pad or a headache with relaxation techniques).

In addition, addressing cultural issues that hinder effective treatment strategies is paramount. Family support is of utmost importance in many cultures, and explaining a psychiatric disorder to family members is difficult and potentially isolating. Finding a health care provider who is sensitive to these potential barriers and able to find effective solutions to ensure that the patient does not feel separated from his or her support system while undergoing treatment will reap the biggest gains.

SUMMARY

Tell me that you don't take that blade and drag it across your skin and pray for the courage to press down.

Girl, Interrupted

It is hoped that emergency providers are no longer tempted by self-injurious behaviors when encountering the difficult patient now that they have been equipped with some strategies to treat both somatizing patients and patients with personality disorders. These stratagems can reduce the number of return visits to the ED, reduce health care costs as well as unnecessary and potentially harmful diagnostic tests to patients, and decrease discord in patient-physician relationships.

REFERENCES

1. Girl Interrupted. 1999. Available at: http://www.imdb.com/character/ch0010009/quotes. Accessed May 22, 2015.
2. Groves JE. Taking care of the taking care of the hateful patient. N Engl J Med 1978;298(16):883–7.
3. World Health Organization. Global status report on non-communicable diseases 2010. Geneva (Switzerland): WHO; 2011.
4. Ottoboni WA. Somatoform disorders. Rosen's emergency medicine concepts and clinical practice. 8th edition. Philadelphia: Saunders; 2014. p. 1481–991.
5. American Psychiatric Association. Diagnostic and statistical manual of mental disorders. 5th edition. Washington, DC: American Psychiatric Publication; 2013.
6. Kirmayer LJ, Groleau D, Looper KJ, et al. Explaining medically unexplained symptoms. Can J Psychiatry 2004;49(10):663–72.
7. Demily C, Sedel F. Psychiatric manifestations of treatable hereditary metabolic disorders in adults. Ann Gen Psychiatry 2014;13:27.
8. Min YW, Rhee PL. Noncardiac chest pain: update on the diagnosis and management. Korean J Gastroenterol 2015;65(2):76–84.
9. Fass R, Achem SR. Noncardiac chest pain: epidemiology, natural course and pathogenesis. J Neurogastroenterol Motil 2011;7:110–23.
10. Krarup AL, Liao D, Gregersen H, et al. Nonspecific motility disorders, irritable esophagus, and chest pain. Ann N Y Acad Sci 2013;1300:96–109.
11. Fass R, Navarro-Rodriguez T. Noncardiac chest pain. J Clin Gastroenterol 2008; 42:636–46.
12. Coss-Adame E, Erdogan A, Rao SS. Treatment of esophageal (noncardiac) chest pain: an expert review. Clin Gastroenterol Hepatol 2014;12:1224–45.
13. Macalpine I, Hunter R. The 'insanity of King George III': a classic case of porphyria. Br Med J 1966;1(5479):65–71.
14. van Dessel N, den Boeft M, van der Wouden JC, et al. Non-pharmacological interventions for somatoform disorders and medically unexplained physical symptoms (MUPS) in adults. Cochrane Database Syst Rev 2014;(11):CD011142.
15. Kumar AR, Katz PO. Functional esophageal disorders: a review of diagnosis and management. Expert Rev Gastroenterol Hepatol 2013;7:453–61.
16. Kleinstäuber M, Witthöft M, Steffanowski A, et al. Pharmacological interventions for somatoform disorders in adults. Cochrane Database Syst Rev 2014;(11):CD010628.
17. Fenyo G. Acute abdominal disease in the elderly: experience from two series in Stockholm. Am J Surg 1982;143(6):751–4.
18. Spangler R, Van Pham T, Khoujah D, et al. Abdominal emergencies in the geriatric patient. Int J Emerg Med 2014;7:43.

19. Crimlisk H. The little imitator—porphyria: a neuropsychiatric disorder. J Neurol Neurosurg Psychiatr 1997;62:319–28.
20. Zijdenbos IL, de Wit NJ, van der Heijden GJ, et al. Psychological treatments for the management of irritable bowel syndrome. Cochrane Database Syst Rev 2009;(1):CD006442.
21. Kompoliti K, Wilson B, Stebbins G, et al. Immediate vs delayed treatment of psychogenic movement disorders with short term psychodynamic psychotherapy: randomized clinical trial. Parkinsonism Relat Disord 2014;20(1):60–3.
22. Dallocchio C, Arbasino C, Klersy C, et al. The effects of physical activity on psychogenic movement disorders. Mov Disord 2010;25(4):421–5.
23. Dallocchio C, Marangi A, Tinazzi M. Functional or psychogenic movement disorders: an endless enigmatic tale. Front Neurol 2015;6:37.
24. Ness D. Physical therapy management for conversion disorder: case series. J Neurol Phys Ther 2007;31(1):30–9.
25. Kanaan RA, Armstrong D, Wessely SC. Neurologists' understanding and management of conversion disorder. J Neurol Neurosurg Psychiatr 2011;82(9):961–6.
26. Garcia-Campayo J, Alda M, Sobradiel N, et al. Personality disorders in somatization disorder patients: a controlled study in Spain. J Psychosom Res 2007;62: 675–80.
27. Strous RD, Ulman AM, Kotler M. The hateful patient revisited: relevance for 21st century medicine. Eur J Intern Med 2006;17(6):387–93.
28. Betan EJ, Kegley Heim A, Zittel Conklin C, et al. Countertransference phenomena and personality pathology in clinical practice: an empirical investigation. Am J Psychiatry 2005;16:890–8.
29. Mason BJ, Quello S, Goodell V, et al. Gabapentin treatment for alcohol dependence: a randomized controlled trial. JAMA Intern Med 2014;174(1):70–7.
30. Lavigne JE, Heckler C, Mathews J, et al. A randomized, controlled, double-blinded clinical trial of gabapentin 300 versus 900 mg versus placebo for anxiety symptoms in breast cancer survivors. Breast Cancer Res Treat 2012;136:479–86.
31. Dowben JS, Grant JS, Froelich KD, et al. Hydroxyzine for anxiety: another look at an old drug. Perspect Psychiatr Care 2013;49:75–7.
32. Tassone DM, Boyce E, Guyer J, et al. Pregabalin: a novel gamma-aminobutyric acid analogue in the treatment of neuropathic pain, partial-onset seizures, and anxiety disorders. Clin Ther 2007;29(1):26–48.
33. Darba J, Kaskens L, Perez C, et al. Pharmacoeconomic outcomes for pregabalin: a systematic review in neuropathic pain, generalized anxiety disorder, and epilepsy from a Spanish perspective. Adv Ther 2014;31:1–29.
34. Fjorback LO, Arendt M, Ornbøl E, et al. Mindfulness therapy for somatization disorder and functional somatic syndromes: randomized trial with one-year follow-up. J Psychosom Res 2013;74(1):31–40.
35. Lazar SW, Bush G, Gollub RL, et al. Functional brain mapping of the relaxation response and meditation. Neuroreport 2000;11(7):1581–5.

Special Considerations in Pediatric Psychiatric Populations

Natalie Pon, MD[a], Bianca Asan, MD[b], Sharadamani Anandan, MD[a],
Alexander Toledo, DO, PharmD[c],*

KEYWORDS

- Autism • ASD • Autism spectrum disorders • ADHD
- Attention deficit hyperactivity disorder • Pediatric • Suicide

KEY POINTS

- Proper treatment of the pediatric psychiatric population can be challenging. Emergency department (ED) boarding, availability of child and adolescent psychiatrists, lack of parental understanding, and inexperience working with children with special needs are just some of the obstacles the ED physician will encounter.
- Suicidal ideation and aggressive or homicidal behavior are the 2 most common pediatric mental health presentations in the ED.
- Children and adolescents with autism spectrum disorder who present with acute behavioral regression that compromises safety should be evaluated using a multidisciplinary approach that includes organic, social, and psychiatric investigations.
- Oppositional-defiant disorder and conduct disorder are common presentations of disruptive behavior in the ED.
- The Internet and social media can have both a positive and negative effect on vulnerable children and adolescents.

INTRODUCTION

The increasing incidence of pediatric psychiatric disorders has been discussed in the literature for more than 2 decades. The 1999 US Surgeon General Report on Mental Health estimates 4 million children and adolescents in this country suffer from a

Disclosures: None.
[a] Department of Psychiatry, Baylor College of Medicine, 1 Baylor Plaza, BCM 350, Houston, TX 77030, USA; [b] Section of Emergency Medicine, Ben Taub Hospital, Baylor College of Medicine, 1504 Taub Loop, Houston, TX 77030, USA; [c] Department of Child Health, University of Arizona College of Medicine, Arizona Children's Center, 2601 East Roosevelt Street, Phoenix, AZ 85008, USA
* Corresponding author.
E-mail address: alexander_toledo@dmgaz.org

Emerg Med Clin N Am 33 (2015) 811–824
http://dx.doi.org/10.1016/j.emc.2015.07.008
0733-8627/15/$ – see front matter © 2015 Elsevier Inc. All rights reserved.

serious mental disorder that causes significant functional impairments at home, at school, and with peers. Half of all lifetime cases of mental disorders begin by age 14 and in any given year, only 20% of children with mental disorders are identified and receive mental health services.[1]

The number of pediatric visits to the emergency department (ED) for psychiatric illness is also increasing.[2] Pediatric mental health visits now make up to 5% of total pediatric ED visits.[3] At our Psychiatry Emergency Center at Ben Taub Hospital (Houston, TX), a Level 1 Trauma Center that provides 24-hour coverage for psychiatric emergencies, a significant increase was seen from 2010 to 2012. Over these 3 years, we saw a sixfold increase of pediatric cases presenting for psychiatric evaluation.

This coupled with a decreased availability of inpatient and outpatient mental health services for children has created a crisis in EDs around the country.[4] The ED boarding of pediatric psychiatric patients also has become commonplace. In one study, the mean ED length of stay of children with psychiatric complaints deemed major was 1127 minutes.[5] This was 7 times longer than a control group with nonpsychiatric complaints in the same study.

Although the ED is a safety net for these patients, the environment itself can be counterproductive. The loud, crowded, and quick-paced ED can be detrimental to children suffering from anxiety, paranoia, or autism.

The ED provider is now obligated to care for this population for extended periods of time. We discuss the risk stratification and interventions necessary when dealing with children and adolescents presenting with suicidal ideation and violent behavior. In addition, we discuss the unique approaches to patients with autism spectrum disorders (ASDs) and attention deficit hyperactivity disorder (ADHD).

TRIAGE OF THE PEDIATRIC EMERGENCY PATIENT

With the increasing number of children presenting to the ED for psychiatric complaints, an effective triage tool is necessary. One study indicated that 40% of pediatric psychiatric ED visits were not urgent. Classification systems, such as the Rosenn urgency classification system, can help ED physicians and psychiatric consults classify need and acuity for psychiatric intervention.[6]

The following is the Rosenn urgency classification system for child and adolescent psychiatric emergencies[6]:

- Class I: Potentially life-threatening emergencies (eg, suicidal and homicidal behavior).
- Class II: States of heightened disturbance requiring urgent intervention (eg, witnessing or being a victim of rape, violence, kidnapping, death of a parent or sibling).
- Class III: Serious conditions requiring prompt but not necessarily immediate intervention (eg, school refusal, verbal threats of suicide or violence, child unmanageable but not dangerous).
- Class IV: Situations in which intervention is demanded but not necessarily psychiatrically warranted (eg, ignorance of proper mental health channels, consumer frustration with overburdened mental health system, interagency struggle, chronic antisocial behavior).

The mental status examination of a child also can help in classifying which cases require more urgent intervention. Observation and assessment of the following areas is necessary[7]:

- Physical appearance
- Manner of relating to examiner and parents

- Ease of separation
- Affect
- Mood
- Orientation to time, place, person
- Content and form of thought, including hallucinations, delusions, thought disorder
- Speech and language
- Overall intelligence, attention, and memory
- Neurologic functioning
- Judgment and insight
- Preferred modes of communication (ie, play, drawing, direct discourse)

DEPRESSION AND SUICIDAL IDEATION

Suicide was the second leading cause of death among children 12 to 17 years of age in 2010.[8] Suicide attempts account for a significant number of ED visits. Although suicidal intent and the long-term risk of death by suicide 10 years after a suicide-related event is approximately 1%, visits to the ED for suicide-related events may be more strongly associated with the intent to die.[9] Although the ratio of suicide attempts to success for ages 15 to 24 is 100 to 200 to 1,[10] the ED physician cannot become nonchalant. Female teenagers are more likely to consider and attempt suicide, but male teenagers are 5 times more likely to be successful. Male adolescents are more likely to use firearms or attempt hanging, whereas female adolescents are more likely attempt to overdose.[11]

Risk factors for attempting suicide include[11]:

- Previous attempts
- Mood and behavioral disorders
- Recent psychiatric hospitalization
- Substance abuse
- Family history of suicide
- Physical or sexual abuse
- Homelessness
- Identification as lesbian, gay, bisexual, or transsexual

PATIENT EVALUATION OVERVIEW

The safety of the patient and staff is paramount. The patient should be placed in an area where they can easily be observed by staff. Preferably the patient should be placed in a gown for easy identification and to limit the possibility of eloping. A search of belongings should be performed to remove any materials that could be used for self-harm. Additionally, removal of communication devices, such as cell phones, may help avoid unnecessary agitation in the patient from phone calls, text messages, or social media. Limiting visitors is also helpful, as romantic and family disputes are a common cause for suicide attempts in adolescents. The room should be cleared of unnecessary cables and supplies that could be used for self-harm.

Physical examination is routine, with special attention to mental status, focal neurologic deficits, and potential toxidromes. Most pediatric patients, especially those with preexisting mental health issues, normal physical examination, vital signs, and mental status often require no further testing. The routine use of laboratory tests for screening in this patient population has been repeatedly shown to be unnecessary.[12,13] One study of an urban pediatric ED found that only 9.1% of patients needed a laboratory workup, and the average charges for laboratory assessments, secondary ambulance transfers, and wages for sitters were $1,241,295 per patient.[13] Unfortunately, many inpatient psychiatric facilities continue to mandate this practice.

Speaking with both the patient and the patient's family is necessary to ascertain the acuity, chronology, and risk to the patient. To facilitate candid discussion, it is recommended that the interviewer meet separately with each. It is also helpful to see the child and parents together to observe their interaction and to assess how they formulate and discuss the problem together.[7] The information gathered from each person involved can be vastly different. Parents are more likely than their children to report disruptive or externalizing behaviors, such as restlessness, inattention, impulsiveness, oppositionality, or aggression. Conversely, children are more likely to report anxious or depressive feelings and symptoms, including suicidal thoughts and acts, of which the parents may be unaware.[7]

Ascertaining psychiatric urgency in the pediatric population is difficult for many ED physicians. The paucity of psychiatric resources in many areas often leaves the ED responsible for triaging these patients. Therefore, understanding which presenting factors are associated with higher acuity is crucial. Edelsohn and colleagues[6] found the following to be independent predictors of urgency in a pediatric population:

- Involuntary arrival status
- Adolescent, risk proportional to age
- Psychosis or affective disorder
- Violent behavior
- Department of Health Services involvement

Adolescents are more likely to engage in making threats, physical aggression, or running away. They are at higher risk for serious emotional disorders, such as depression and schizophrenia, than preadolescents.[6] Adolescents will often minimize their symptoms and intent citing a desire to go to sleep and "not thinking" when asked about their actions.[11] It is crucial to take the risk factors listed previously into account, as well expressions of hopelessness and impulsivity. Protective factors that may influence the desire to attempt suicide include religious belief and concern not to hurt family.[14]

PHARMACOLOGIC TREATMENT

The initiation of therapy by an ED physician is not recommended. No pharmacologic agent is indicated to specifically treat suicidal ideation. Furthermore, the agents most often prescribed for depression and anxiety, selective serotonin reuptake inhibitors, carry a risk of increasing suicidal ideation and must be closely monitored.[11] Supportive care is otherwise advised.

DISPOSITION

The overall rate for pediatric psychiatric admissions in one study was 23.4%, with the rate increasing to 58.3% when limited to ages 15 to 17 years.[15] There are no validated criteria to risk stratify the suicidal pediatric patient. General consensus seems to agree that the following require immediate referral for inpatient psychiatric placement[11]:

- Continued desire to die
- Severe hopelessness
- Ongoing agitation
- Inability to engage in a discussion around safety planning
- Inadequate support system/ability to adequate monitoring and follow-up
- High lethality attempt or an attempt with clear expectation of death

Occasionally one will encounter the patient who requires involuntary admission or the parents who do not consent to psychiatric placement. Each state has its own laws regarding involuntary commitment. The ED provider should become familiar with local laws and protocols.

Special care must be taken with those pediatric patients who will be discharged home. Lack of finances, limited community resources, and accessibility of mental health providers can hinder the patient's ability to follow up. Consultation with a social worker and discussion with the primary care provider may help avoid these pitfalls and uncover options not previously known to the ED provider.[11]

THE AGGRESSIVE OR VIOLENT PEDIATRIC PATIENT

Pediatric psychiatric patients exhibiting dangerous behaviors, which include threatening staff, threatening other patients, aggressive behavior, violence, and elopement have been well reported.[3,16] In one study of patients with problematic behaviors, almost half required chemical and/or physical restraints in the ED. Risk factors for violence behaviors in the ED were those presenting with a complaint of aggressive behavior, with a psychiatric or a history of previous psychiatric hospitalization. There was no association between dangerous behaviors and sex, age, or use of psychiatric medications.[17]

General Guidelines for Treatment of Agitation

The most critical step in treating agitation or aggression is determining the underlying cause. The workup includes review of psychiatric history, assessment of pain, evaluation of substance intoxication or withdrawal, medication interaction or side effects, metabolic abnormalities, sleep deprivation, hypoxia, sepsis, trauma, or an acute or chronic medical illness. All may be associated with behavioral instability and must be fully explored to determine effective intervention.[18]

The patient with escalating behavior may progress through the following 4 stages[19]:

1. Verbal stage: the patient may use nonspecific threats and abusive language toward others.
2. Motor stage: the patient remains in constant motion, agitated and often pacing.
3. Property damage stage: the patient proceeds to destroy equipment in the room.
4. Attack stage: the patient attempts to inflict harm on self or others.

The least invasive means of deescalation is always preferred. Creating a safe, comfortable environment, listening attentively, and speaking calmly often suffice. **Box 1** describes recommendations for creating a safe environment and encouraging communication.

TREATMENT

The treatment of acute agitation in the pediatric population is based on several factors. The patient's response to verbal cues and the perceived risk of the child causing harm to himself or herself or others will often guide therapy. The overall goal is to provide a safe environment for the child and staff while providing adequate anxiolysis for the patient. Interventions can be escalated based on perceived response; however, it is recommended that the least-invasive intervention possible be used. Pharmacologic restraint should be used sparingly and with lowest possible dose to achieve the desired effect. **Box 2** lists recommendations for incorporation of pharmacologic interventions and **Table 1** describes commonly used agents for agitation in the pediatric population.

Box 1
General guidelines for treatment of agitation

Patient

- Remove access to breakable objects/equipment.
- Reduce environmental stimulation (dim lights, reduce noise, minimize visitors, redirect traffic near room).
- Clearly introduce yourself, assure patient that you are there to keep him/her safe; this is your job.
- Use simple language, soft voice, and slow movements.
- Use relaxed body language.
- Stay 3–4 feet away from the patient.
- Address hunger, thirst, comfort, warmth.
- Explain what is to come next. Discuss restraints and offer reward for calmer behavior.
- Listen and empathize (a treatment cornerstone).
- Tell child how you plan to honor his or her reasonable requests.
- Find things for the child to control, like choice of drinks.
- Remain engaged; perceived ignoring may encourage escalations.
- Offer distracting toys/sensory modalities.
- Clarify the child's goal and then try to link his or her cooperation to that goal.
- Maintain privacy and respect, a nonjudgmental attitude.
- Remember not to take their anger personally.

Family and Staff

- Ask caregiver or patient about why he or she is upset and offer ways to calm the patient.
- Engage consultants: security, social work, psychiatry.
- Prepare with staff for the next step if the calming strategies fail.
- Prepare an algorithm for pharmacologic management if the listed methods fail, including attention to the clinical situation, preexisting medications, intoxication status, medical history, allergies.

From Cummings MR, Miller BD. Pharmacologic management of behavioral instability in medically ill pediatric patients. Curr Opin Pediatr 2004;16(5):516–22; and Sorrentino A. Chemical restraints for the agitated, violent, or psychotic pediatric patient in the emergency department: controversies and recommendations. Curr Opin Pediatr 2004;16(2):201–5.

Definitions for Reference

- Restraint: The involuntary immobilization of a person through the use of chemical, physical, or mechanical means.
- Chemical restraint: A drug used as a restraint is a medication used to control behavior or to restrict a patient's freedom of movement and is not standard treatment for the patient's medical or psychiatric condition. Chemical restraint is different from the ongoing use of medication for the treatment of symptoms of underlying psychiatric illness.
- Mechanical restraint: Use of leather or cloth restraints, papoose board, calming blanket, body carrier, and other implements used in restraint procedures.

Box 2

General emergency pharmacology guidelines

If patient is already on psychotropic medications, consider dosing those if possible, unless there is suspicion of toxicity.

- Offer oral medication first.
- If not at usual dose time, consider one-fourth to one-half of total daily amount as a single dose.
- Check maximum dose range.
- Avoid aripiprazole due to potential for agitation.

Delirium present: treat underlying medical derangement.

- Avoid benzodiazepines if there is evidence of depressant intoxication.

Symptom-specific medication.

- Anxiety: Lorazepam, consider diphenhydramine.
- Mania or psychotic thoughts: haloperidol, risperidone, olanzapine, ziprasidone.
- Impulsive, maladaptive aggression: risperidone or olanzapine.
- General agitation: can give benzodiazepine or antipsychotic. One can mix haloperidol and lorazepam in the same syringe. With other antipsychotics, can add benzodiazepine after 30 minutes if needed.

From Cummings MR, Miller BD. Pharmacologic management of behavioral instability in medically ill pediatric patients. Curr Opin Pediatr 2004;16(5):516–22; and Sorrentino A. Chemical restraints for the agitated, violent, or psychotic pediatric patient in the emergency department: controversies and recommendations. Curr Opin Pediatr 2004;16(2):201–5.

- Physical restraint: Restraint that involves one or more staff members in bodily contact with the patient and does not use a mechanical apparatus.
- Seclusion: The involuntary confinement of a person in a room alone so that the person is physically prevented from leaving.

Restraint Specifications for Children per Latest Guidelines

- The American Academy of Child and Adolescent Psychiatry practice parameters indicate 3 levels of crisis management[20]:
  - Level 1, or nonrestrictive interventions, such as verbal prompting and deescalating.
  - Level 2, or restrictive interventions, such as ignoring behavior ("extinction") and room restriction.
  - Level 3, or the most restrictive interventions, such as seclusion, physical restraint (children), mechanical restraint (adolescents), and chemical restraint, all of which produce both the most external control over an individual's behavior coupled with the greatest limitation on his or her autonomy. In these cases, the risk of harm to the patient and/or others outweighs considerations of promoting his or her autonomy.

The only indications for the use of seclusion and restraint are the following:

- Prevent dangerous behavior to self or others.
- Prevent disorganization or serious disruption of the treatment program, including serious damage to property.

Table 1
Pharmacologic treatment of the agitated pediatric patient

Medication	Dose and Route	Prepubertal	Pubertal	Pharmacokinetics
Haloperidol	0.025–0.075 mg/kg/dose PO/IM May repeat PO every 60 min, IM every 20–30 min	0.5–2 mg PO/IM	2–5 mg PO/IM	Onset: PO 60 min, IM 20–30 min Peak concentration: PO 2–6 h, IM 20 min Duration: 4 h
Diphenhydramine	1 mg/kg PO/IM/IV May repeat PO every 20–30 min, IM every 20 min × 2–4	25–50 mg PO/IM	50–100 mg PO/IM	Onset: PO 15 min to 1 h Peak concentration: PO 2–4 h Duration: 4–6 h Limited data on IM Onset 10–15 min
Lorazepam	0.05 mg/kg PO/IM/IV May repeat PO every 20–30 min, IM every 15–20 min	0.5–2 mg PO/IM	1–2 mg PO/IM	Onset: PO 20–30 min, IM 15 min Peak concentration: 0.5–3 h Duration: 6–8 h PO or IM
Olanzapine	0.1 mg/kg PO/IM May repeat PO every 30–45 min, IM every 20–30 min × 1	2.5 mg PO/IM	5–10 mg PO/IM	Onset: Limited data PO 20–30 min, IM 10–20 min Peak concentration: IM 15–45 min Duration: 24 h
Risperidone	0.025–0.05 mg/kg PO May repeat PO every 60 min × 2–4	0.25–0.5 mg PO	0.5–1 mg PO	Onset: PO 30 min Peak concentration: 1–2 h

Abbreviations: IM, intramuscular; IV, intravenous; PO, oral.
Adapted from Adimando AJ, Poncin YB, Baum CR. Pharmacologic management of the agitated pediatric patient. Pediatr Emerg Care 2010;26(11):856–60.

- Measures promoting the child's self-control or less restrictive options have failed or are impractical.

Pharmacologic Strategies

The frequency with which physical or chemical restraint of a child is necessary in an ED is mostly unknown; one report reveals some form of restraint (physical, chemical, or both) was used for 6.8% of all child and adolescent psychiatric evaluations.[21] Pharmacologic intervention should not be used as punishment for the patient or as convenience for the staff. The aim is to get the patient calmed, not sedated.

The following factors affect hospitalization for agitation[22]:

- Type and severity of the psychiatric disorder
- Family's level of distress
- Level of parental capacity to contain the child (inverse relationship)

AUTISM SPECTRUM DISORDERS AND ATTENTION DEFICIT HYPERACTIVITY DISORDER
INTRODUCTION

ADHD and autism are common conditions among the pediatric population. They can overlap with acute organic processes or coexist with a broad spectrum of psychiatric conditions. Mechanisms underlying these disorders are poorly understood and are multifactorial in nature. A holistic approach combined with pharmacologic therapy in very specific circumstances has shown to be more successful compared with pharmacologic treatment alone.

The existence of a broad spectrum of manifestations and the considerable rate of coexistence with other pathologies necessitate a personalized approach. Family is a very important source of information to understand the baseline behavior of the patients.

PATIENT EVALUATION OVERVIEW
Autism

Autism is the core disorder of the pervasive developmental disorders. It may be evident before the age of 3 years and is characterized by impairments in communication and social interaction, the presence of restricted and repetitive behaviors, and impaired imagination.[23] One in every 68 US children has been identified as being on the autism pervasive disorder spectrum.[24]

In one study, 80% of children with ASD were found to have at least one psychiatric comorbidity.[25] Unnecessary referrals and the lack of availability of specialized care for these patients has led to an increase of ED visits for psychiatric complaints. Although these children can present for the usual illnesses of childhood, one study found that visits of children with ASD were more likely to be for psychiatric reasons compared with visits of children without ASD (12.9% vs 1.75%).[26]

Associated presentations

- Externalizing: Externalizing behaviors are thought to be the leading cause for psychiatric visits among children with ASD.[27] This may result in behavioral crises involving physical aggression, disruptive behavior, and self-injury. Internalizing behavior can be a huge obstacle for the child who is experiencing them. As a result, internalizing behaviors often go unrecognized until the child begins to engage in externalizing behavior.

- Psychotic disorders: Children with ASD and high autistic trait scores are more likely to have psychotic experiences. Autism and psychotic disorders have historically been considered related diagnostic entities. High rates of idiosyncratic fears, anxiety reactions, and thought disorder are thought to increase the risk of psychosis.[28] Additionally, neurodevelopmental disorders that typically manifest in childhood (such as autism) or in young adulthood (such as schizophrenia) share overlapping pathogenic mechanisms linked with perturbation in brain development.[29] Children and adolescents with ASD are more likely to exhibit psychotic features in the ED than their counterparts without ASD. ED physicians may misinterpret a complex psychiatric presentation that consists of cognitive and social issues with psychosis.[26]

Behavioral interventions

Children with autism may not respond to the usual deescalation techniques used by ED staff. Hypersensitivity to sensory input, impaired social and cognitive skills, and limited ability to communicate all contribute the patient's anxiety.

Language

Children with autism often interpret language literally. Unambiguous, clear phrasing in short sentences is helpful. Probing and clarifying the meaning behind the reported psychotic experiences is important when assessing these experiences.

Attention Deficit Hyperactivity Disorder

ADHD, also called hyperkinetic disorder, is a neurodevelopmental disorder characterized by high levels of inattention, hyperactivity, and impulsive behavior. It is usually first diagnosed in childhood and often remains into adulthood.[30,31] Younger patients with ADHD frequently present to EDs with crises involving behavioral dyscontrol; legal, school, or family conflict; and substance abuse.[32] These children's lives are marked by impulsivity, self-defeating behavior, and dysphoria or depression.[33]

Associated presentations

- Suicide attempts: ADHD is associated with an increased risk of both attempted and completed suicide. It is postulated that they may not have frequent parasuicidal presentations before completion.[33] A high prevalence of conflicts between parents and the child, trauma victimization, social impairment, conduct disorder, and depression have been found in this population.[34] The prevalence of ADHD in one series of patients referred after ED visit for suicidal ideation or attempt was 25.6% for children younger than 12 years and 5.7% for those age 12 to 18 years.[35]
- Deliberate self-poisoning (DSP) and deliberate self-harm (DSH): ADHD is associated with a higher incidence of ED visits for DSP and DSH. DSP and DSH relate to nonlethal self-injurious behavior and is much more common than actualized suicide.[36] In one series of children (younger than 12 years) presenting for DSH, the incidence of ADHD was 43.2%.[35] An accurate evaluation of the psychiatric status of patients with ADHD is critical for preventing DSP events.[37]
- Hallucinations: Both the use of methylphenidate and ADHD itself have been associated with nonpsychotic hallucinations.[38] In one series, 22% of patients presenting with nonpsychotic hallucinations to pediatric psychiatric emergency service had ADHD.[39]
- Comorbidities: ADHD is associated with several harmful behaviors and disorders.[35]

- ○ Increased incidence of traumatic injury
- ○ Increased risk of addiction
- ○ Increased incidence of violent behavior
- ○ Increased risk of being a victim of sexual abuse
- ○ High incidence of comorbid bipolar disorder
- ○ Higher risk of having an eating disorder

OPPOSITIONAL-DEFIANT DISORDER AND CONDUCT DISORDER

The ED physician is also likely to encounter patients who present with exacerbations of behavioral disorders. Of those presenting to the ED with a diagnosis, oppositional-defiant disorder (ODD) and conduct disorder (CD) are most frequently encountered. These children are often referred directly by the school to the ED or are brought in by parents who are overwhelmed and frustrated by the patient's conduct. However, many of these patients do not present primarily for their behavioral problems. In one series of children presenting to the ED with behavioral disorders in Canada, the investigators found that 45.8% had a primary complaint of depression or self-harm and 28.8% were evaluated for violent behavior.[40]

These children are vulnerable to adverse social repercussions, secondary psychiatric conditions, and poor decision making. They are cited as being less popular among peers, and having higher rates of depression, suicide attempts, and anxiety. They are also more likely to engage in risk taking, substance abuse, and interactions with law enforcement.[40]

ODD is a mental disorder arising in childhood that is characterized by persistent angry, irritable, argumentative, negativistic, hostile, and defiant behavior toward authority figures.[39,40] Although such behaviors are common in children, in ODD the behaviors occur at particularly high levels, ultimately interfering with functioning. CD is a more concerning mental disorder arising in childhood associated with high levels of aggression to people or animals, destruction of property, deceitfulness or theft, and serious rule-violating behavior.[40,41] A subset of patients with CD, those with limited prosocial emotions or callous-unemotional traits, carry an especially poor prognosis and are resistant to treatment.[40] These patients exhibit reduced guilt, callousness, uncaring behavior, and reduced empathy.[40] ED treatment of these disorders is limited to management of secondary presentations and treatment of acute agitation and aggression, as previously discussed.

EFFECT OF SOCIAL MEDIA AND INTERNET ON PEDIATRIC PSYCHIATRIC PRESENTATIONS

With the advent of the Internet and, specifically, social media, a new source of influence has been introduced to youth. The increased availability and decreased cost of cell phones and Internet service have made access to social media almost universal. Ninety-four percent of teens have a computer or have access to one, 63% go online daily, and 36% are online several times a day.[42] Adolescents have reported an average of approximately 1.7 hours of computer use per day, and 53% of those 15 to 18 years old reported visiting social networking sites on a typical day.[42] This has given rise to several new problems and exacerbated old ones facing pediatric patients. These include, but are not limited to, Internet addiction, body image disorders, pornography addiction, cyberbullying, and suicide.[42,43] The latter 2 deserve special attention and are especially relevant to the previously discussed topics.

Cyberbullying has been defined as the collective label used to define forms of bullying that use electronic means such as the Internet and mobile phones to aggressively and intentionally harm someone.[44] The incidence of cyberbullying among adolescents has been reported to range from 15% to 40%.[42] Although some studies suggest a link between cyberbullying and increased risk of self-harm, suicidal ideation, and suicide attempts for both offenders and victims, there are conflicting data.[42,45] Research also suggests that cyberbullying may have a more negative impact than traditional methods of bullying.[45] Once suicidal thoughts or ideation is present, social media and the Internet can provide the necessary stimulus to push a patient to an attempt. The presence of prosuicide chat rooms and forums, the availability of "how-to" Web pages, and the effect of media contagion all can affect this vulnerable population.[43] However, research also suggests the Internet and social media are most commonly used by adolescents for constructive reasons, such as seeking support and coping strategies.[46]

SUMMARY

The frequency of pediatric patients presenting to the ED for psychiatric problems is increasing. The ED continues to be a suboptimal place for many of these patients but is often used given the lack of community resources. Suicidal ideation and aggressive behavior will continue to be the most commonly presenting complaints for which urgent attention and intervention are required. Children with autism and ADHD are at especially prone to psychiatric comorbidities and require a specialized approach. Therefore, the ED provider must be familiar with these different pathologies, the resources available to them, and the appropriate treatment for acute exacerbations.

REFERENCES

1. US Department of Health and Human Services. Mental health: a report of the Surgeon General—executive summary. Rockville (MD): US Department of Health and Human Services. Substance Abuse and Mental Health Services Administration, Center for Mental Health Services, National Institutes of Health, National Institute of Mental Health; 1999. p. 8.
2. Ting SA, Sullivan AF, Boudreaux ED, et al. Trends in US emergency department visits for attempted suicide and self-inflicted injury, 1993–2008. Gen Hosp Psychiatry 2012;34(5):557–65.
3. Grupp-Phelan J, Harman JS, Kelleher KJ. Trends in mental health and chronic condition visits by children presenting for care at US emergency departments. Public Health Rep 2007;122(1):55.
4. American Academy of Pediatrics, American College of Emergency Physicians, & Pediatric Emergency Medicine Committee. Pediatric mental health emergencies in the emergency medical services system. Pediatrics 2006;118(4):1764–7.
5. Waseem M, Prasankumar R, Pagan K, et al. A retrospective look at length of stay for pediatric psychiatric patients in an urban emergency department. Pediatr Emerg Care 2011;27(3):170–3.
6. Edelsohn GA, Braitman LE, Rabinovich H, et al. Predictors of urgency in a pediatric psychiatric emergency service. J Am Acad Child Adolesc Psychiatry 2003; 42(10):1197–202.
7. King RA. Practice parameters for the psychiatric assessment of children and adolescents. J Am Acad Child Adolesc Psychiatry 1997;36(10):4S–20S.
8. Perou R, Bitsko RH, Blumberg SJ, et al. Mental health surveillance among children—United States, 2005–2011. MMWR Surveill Summ 2013;62(Suppl 2): 1–35.

9. Newton AS, Hamm MP, Bethell J, et al. Pediatric suicide-related presentations: a systematic review of mental health care in the emergency department. Ann Emerg Med 2010;56(6):649–59.

10. Drapeau CW, McIntosh JL, for the American Association of Suicidology. U.S.A. suicide 2012: official final data. Washington, DC: American Association of Suicidology; 2014. Available at: http://www.suicidology.org. Accessed October 18, 2014.

11. Chun TH, Katz ER, Duffy SJ, et al. Challenges of managing pediatric mental health crises in the emergency department. Child Adolesc Psychiatr Clin N Am 2015;24(1):21–40.

12. Donofrio JJ, Santillanes G, McCammack BD, et al. Clinical utility of screening laboratory tests in pediatric psychiatric patients presenting to the emergency department for medical clearance. Ann Emerg Med 2014;63(6):666–75.

13. Santillanes G, Donofrio JJ, Lam CN, et al. Is medical clearance necessary for pediatric psychiatric patients? J Emerg Med 2014;46(6):800–7.

14. Birmaher B, Brent D, AACAP Work Group on Quality Issues. Practice parameter for the assessment and treatment of children and adolescents with depressive disorders. J Am Acad Child Adolesc Psychiatry 2007;46(11):1503–26.

15. Huffman LC, Wang NE, Saynina O, et al. Predictors of hospitalization after an emergency department visit for California youths with psychiatric disorders. Psychiatr Serv 2012;63(9):896–905.

16. Ryan EP, Hart VS, Messick DL, et al. A prospective study of assault against staff by youths in a state psychiatric hospital. Psychiatr Serv 2014;55(6):665–70.

17. Hilt R. Agitation treatment for pediatric emergency patients. J Am Acad Child Adolesc Psychiatry 2008;47(2):132–8.

18. Cummings MR, Miller BD. Pharmacologic management of behavioral instability in medically ill pediatric patients. Curr Opin Pediatr 2004;16(5):516–22.

19. Sorrentino A. Chemical restraints for the agitated, violent, or psychotic pediatric patient in the emergency department: controversies and recommendations. Curr Opin Pediatr 2004;16(2):201–5.

20. Masters KJ, Bellonci C. Practice parameter for the prevention and management of aggressive behavior in child and adolescent psychiatric institutions, with special reference to seclusion and restraint. J Am Acad Child Adolesc Psychiatry 2002;41(2):4S–25S.

21. Dorfman DH, Mehta SD. Restraint use for psychiatric patients in the pediatric emergency department. Pediatr Emerg Care 2006;22(1):7–12.

22. Golubchik P, Sever J, Finzi-Dottan R, et al. The factors influencing decision making on children's psychiatric hospitalization: a retrospective chart review. Community Ment Health J 2013;49(1):73–8.

23. Oono IP, Honey EJ, McConachie H. Parent-mediated early intervention for young children with autism spectrum disorders (ASD). Cochrane Database Syst Rev 2013;8(6):2380–479.

24. McCarthy M. Autism diagnoses in the US rise by 30%, CDC reports. BMJ 2014; 348:g2520.

25. de Bruin EI, Ferdinand RF, Meester S, et al. High rates of psychiatric co-morbidity in PDD-NOS. J Autism Dev Disord 2007;37(5):877–86.

26. Kalb LG, Stuart EA, Freedman B, et al. Psychiatric-related emergency department visits among children with an autism spectrum disorder. Pediatr Emerg Care 2012;28(12):1269–76.

27. Siegel M, Gabriels RL. Psychiatric hospital treatment of children with autism and serious behavioral disturbance. Child Adolesc Psychiatr Clin N Am 2014;23(1):125–42.

28. Kyriakopoulos M, Stringaris A, Manolesou S, et al. Determination of psychosis-related clinical profiles in children with autism spectrum disorders using latent class analysis. Eur Child Adolesc Psychiatry 2015;24(3):301–7.

29. Owen MJ, O'Donovan MC, Thapar A, et al. Neurodevelopmental hypothesis of schizophrenia. Br J Psychiatry 2011;198(3):173–5.

30. American Psychiatric Association (APA). Diagnostic and statistical manual of mental disorders. 4th edition. Washington, DC: American Psychiatric Association; 1994.

31. World Health Organization (WHO). The ICD-10 classification of mental and behavior disorders. Geneva (Switzerland): WHO; 1992.

32. Klykylo KT, Klykylo WM. Managing attention deficit hyperactivity disorder in the emergency department. Psychiatry (Edgmont) 2008;5(8):43.

33. Harpin VA. The effect of ADHD on the life of an individual, their family, and community from preschool to adult life. Arch Dis Child 2005;90(Suppl 1):i2–7.

34. Impey M, Heun R. Completed suicide, ideation and attempt in attention deficit hyperactivity disorder. Acta Psychiatr Scand 2012;125(2):93–102.

35. Reinhardt MC, Reinhardt CA. Attention deficit-hyperactivity disorder, comorbidities, and risk situations. J Pediatr 2013;89(2):124–30.

36. Ben-Yehuda A, Aviram S, Govezensky J, et al. Suicidal behavior in minors–diagnostic differences between children and adolescents. J Dev Behav Pediatr 2012; 33(7):542–7.

37. Chou IC, Lin CC, Sung FC, et al. Attention-deficit hyperactivity disorder increases the risk of deliberate self-poisoning: a population-based cohort. Eur Psychiatry 2014;29(8):523–7.

38. Edelsohn GA. Hallucinations in children and adolescents: considerations in the emergency setting. Am J Psychiatry 2006;163(5):781–5.

39. Edelsohn GA, Rabinovich H, Portnoy R. Hallucinations in nonpsychotic children. Ann N Y Acad Sci 2003;1008(1):261–4.

40. Liu S, Ali S, Rosychuk RJ, et al. Characteristics of children and youth who visit the emergency department for a behavioural disorder. J Can Acad Child Adolesc Psychiatry 2014;23(2):111.

41. Blair RJR, Leibenluft E, Pine DS. Conduct disorder and callous–unemotional traits in youth. N Engl J Med 2014;371(23):2207–16.

42. Bailin A, Milanaik R, Adesman A. Health implications of new age technologies for adolescents: a review of the research. Curr Opin Pediatr 2014;26(5):605–19.

43. Luxton DD, June JD, Fairall JM. Social media and suicide: a public health perspective. Am J Public Health 2012;102(S2):S195–200.

44. Price M, Dalgleish J. Cyberbullying: experiences, impacts and coping strategies as described by Australian young people. Youth Stud Aust 2010;29(2):51.

45. Van Geel M, Vedder P, Tanilon J. Relationship between peer victimization, cyberbullying, and suicide in children and adolescents: a meta-analysis. JAMA Pediatr 2014;168(5):435–42.

46. Daine K, Hawton K, Singaravelu V, et al. The power of the Web: a systematic review of studies of the influence of the Internet on self-harm and suicide in young people. PLoS One 2013;8(10):e77555.

Psychiatric Emergencies in the Elderly

Veronica Sikka, MD, PhD, MHA, MPH[a,b,*], S. Kalra, MD, MPH[c],
Galwankar Sagar, DNB, MPH, Diplomat. ABEM[a]

KEYWORDS

- Geriatric psychiatric emergencies • Elderly • Dementia • Abuse
- Psychiatric emergencies • Depression • Delirium • NPH

KEY POINTS

- Over the last few decades, there has been a constant increase in the number of geriatric patients visiting the emergency department.
- Besides correct diagnosis, it is important the clinician provide elderly patients with appropriate resources for admission or discharge.
- Resources also often extend to the patients' families, but diagnosis and having a broad differential diagnosis to identify a potentially serious underlying psychiatric emergency in the elderly population is the first, vital step.
- Diagnosis and treatment of geriatric patients can be particularly challenging, given the associated medical comorbidities, polypharmacy, and underlying psychosocial issues that do not make for a straightforward diagnosis and management.

INTRODUCTION

"I can see the words hanging in front of me and I can't reach them, and I don't know who I am, and I don't know what I'm going to lose next," says Alice Howland, the main character in the 2015 film *Still Alice* that highlights the reality of progressive Alzheimer disease and its emergent manifestations. In 2012, the number of people older than 65 years was 43.1 million, composing about 13.7% of the total population. By 2050, the population of Americans 65 years and older is expected to be nearly 87 million and will compose nearly 21% of the total population. This number represents a 147% increase in the geriatric age group compared with a mere 49% increase in the population younger than 65 years.[1] Over the last few decades, there has been a constant increase in the number of geriatric patients

Disclosures: none.
[a] Orlando VA Medical Center Emergency Medicine, Richmond, VA, USA; [b] Emergency Medicine, UCF School of Medicine, Orlando, FL, USA; [c] Department of Research and Innovation, St Luke's University Health Network, Bethlehem, PA, USA
* Corresponding author. 13800 Veterans Way, Orlando, FL 32827.
E-mail address: Veronica.Sikka@va.gov

Emerg Med Clin N Am 33 (2015) 825–839
http://dx.doi.org/10.1016/j.emc.2015.07.009
0733-8627/15/$ – see front matter Published by Elsevier Inc.

visiting the emergency department (ED). According to the 2011 Centers for Disease Control and Prevention National Hospital Ambulatory Medical Care Survey, almost 15% of total ED visits comprised patients 65 years and older.[2] Diagnosis and treatment of these patients can be particularly challenging given the associated medical comorbidities, polypharmacy, and underlying psychosocial issues that do not make for a straightforward diagnosis and management. This review article identifies common psychiatric emergencies among the geriatric population and its associated management.

DELIRIUM

According to the *Diagnostic and Statistical Manual of Mental Disorders* (Fourth Edition) (*DSM-IV*) criteria, delirium is an acute disturbance of consciousness with decreased attention, change in cognition, or development of perceptual disturbance that develops over a short period of time with diurnal fluctuations and evidence that the disturbance is caused by a general medical condition, substance abuse or withdrawal, or multiple causes. Although delirium is a common psychiatric emergency that affects an estimated 30% to 50% of hospitalized elderly patients,[3] delirium still poses significant diagnostic challenges with nondetection rates as high as 70%.

The onset of delirium is normally rapid with fluctuations in consciousness. The patient history is very helpful in ascertaining sudden changes in cognition that are perhaps related to underlying medical conditions (ie, urinary tract infection [UTI], recent fall), medication use, and risk of withdrawal from drugs or alcohol. Delirium can be categorized into 3 subtypes: hyperactive, hypoactive, and mixed.[4] Patients with hyperactive delirium present very hypervigilant, restless, or agitated and can complain of auditory or visual hallucinations. The hypoactive form of delirium is associated with increased lethargy, somnolence, and dulled psychomotor function. This form of delirium is often overlooked by clinicians and mistaken for depression.[5] Finally, mixed delirium is associated with features of both hyperactive and hypoactive types.

Tools that can be used in the ED include the Confusion Assessment Method (CAM), which is a short, standardized diagnostic algorithm of delirium and the Memorial Delirium Assessment (MDA) scale, which can be used to quantify the severity of the delirium. CAM includes 2 parts. Part 1 is an assessment instrument that screens for overall cognitive impairment. Part 2 includes only those 4 features that were found to have the greatest ability to distinguish delirium or reversible confusion from other types of cognitive impairment. The tool can be administered in less than 5 minutes. It closely correlates with the *DSM-IV* criteria for delirium. **Boxes 1** and **2** list the CAM instrument and diagnostic algorithm.

The MDA scale is a 10-item, 4-point, clinician-rated scale that is designed to quantify the severity of delirium. **Fig. 1** lists the 10 questions associated with the MDA.

MDA total scores differ significantly between patients with delirium and those with other cognitive impairment disorders or no cognitive impairment. It is also used for making the diagnosis of delirium, and a cutoff score of 13 has been shown to be useful for making the diagnosis of delirium.[6] In a fairly robust study that compared assessment scales for delirium, it was found that the CAM is the most useful instrument in terms of its accuracy, brevity, and ease of use by clinicians and lay interviewers.[7]

Managing delirium implies identifying and managing the underlying cause. Environmental interventions, such as noise reduction, proper illumination, stimulus modification, cueing, and reassurance, are integral parts of delirium treatment.[8] If patients' safety and ability to participate in medical management is compromised, pharmacologic interventions may be required. Most evidence supports the use of low-dose haloperidol, with higher doses being associated with adverse effects.[9]

Box 1
CAM instrument

1. Acute onset: Is there evidence of an acute change in mental status from the patient's baseline?

2A. Inattention: Did the patient have difficulty focusing attention, for example, being easily distractible or having difficulty keeping track of what was being said?

2B. If present or abnormal: Did this behavior fluctuate during the interview, that is, tend to come and go or increase and decrease in severity?

3. Disorganized thinking: Was the patient's thinking disorganized or incoherent, such as rambling or irrelevant conversation, unclear or illogical flow of ideas, or unpredictable switching from subject to subject?

4. Altered level of consciousness: Overall, how would you rate this patient's level of consciousness? (Alert [normal]; vigilant [hyperalert, overly sensitive to environmental stimuli, startled very easily]; lethargic [drowsy, easily aroused]; stupor [difficult to arouse]; coma [unarousable]; uncertain)

5. Disorientation: Was the patient disoriented at any time during the interview, such as thinking that he or she was somewhere other than the hospital, using the wrong bed, or misjudging the time of day?

6. Memory impairment: Did the patient demonstrate any memory problems during the interview, such as inability to remember events in the hospital or difficulty remembering instructions?

7. Perceptual disturbances: Did the patient have any evidence of perceptual disturbances, for example, hallucinations, illusions, or misinterpretations (such as thinking something was moving when it was not)?

8A. Psychomotor agitation: At any time during the interview, did the patient have an unusually increased level of motor activity, such as restlessness, picking at bedclothes, tapping fingers, or making frequent sudden changes of position?

8B. Psychomotor retardation: At any time during the interview did the patient have an unusually decreased level of motor activity, such as sluggishness, staring into space, staying in one position for a long time, or moving very slowly?

9. Altered sleep-wake cycle: Did the patient have evidence of disturbance of the sleep-wake cycle, such as excessive daytime sleepiness with insomnia at night?

From Inouye S, van Dyck C, Alessi C, et al. Clarifying confusion: the confusion assessment method. Ann Intern Med 1990;113(12):941–8. © 2003 Sharon K. Inouye, MD, MPH.

DEMENTIA

Dementia is a common neuropsychiatric syndrome associated with progressive decline in function across multiple cognitive domains. It affects anywhere from 8% to 10% of people older than 65 years and nearly 50% of those older than 85 years.[10] Alzheimer disease is the most common cause of dementia followed by vascular dementia and dementia with Lewy bodies. About 80% of patients with dementia experience some form of behavioral or psychological symptoms of dementia (BPSD). These symptoms include agitation and aggression, delusions, hallucinations and misidentifications, screaming and repetitive vocalizations, circadian rhythm dysregulation, and wandering.

The first step in evaluating behavioral disturbance in patients with dementia is to assess for medical, pharmacologic, and environmental variables that may have precipitated the behavior. Possible causes of BPSD[11] are listed in **Box 3**.

Box 2
The CAM diagnostic algorithm

Feature 1: Acute-onset and fluctuating course

This feature is usually obtained from a family member or nurse and is shown by positive responses to the following questions: Is there evidence of an acute change in mental status from the patient's baseline? Did the (abnormal) behavior fluctuate during the day, that is, tend to come and go or increase and decrease in severity?

Feature 2: Inattention

This feature is shown by a positive response to the following question: Did the patient have difficulty focusing attention, for example, being easily distractible or having difficulty keeping track of what was being said?

Feature 3: Disorganized thinking

This feature is shown by a positive response to the following question: Was the patient's thinking disorganized or incoherent, such as rambling or irrelevant conversation, unclear or illogical flow of ideas, or unpredictable switching from subject to subject?

Feature 4: Altered level of consciousness

This feature is shown by any answer other than *alert* to the following question:

Overall, how would you rate this patient's level of consciousness? (alert [normal], vigilant [hyperalert], lethargic [drowsy, easily aroused], stupor [difficult to arouse], or coma [unarousable]).

The diagnosis of delirium by CAM requires the presence of features 1 and 2 and either 3 or 4.
 From Inouye S, van Dyck C, Alessi C, et al. Clarifying confusion: the confusion assessment method. Ann Intern Med 1990;113(12):941–8. © 2003 Sharon K. Inouye, MD, MPH.

Diagnosis can be challenging given the fluctuating nature of the symptoms and the patients' impeded ability to communicate. Validated and reliable scales, such as the Behavioral Pathology in Alzheimer disease Rating Scale or the Cohen-Mansfield Agitation Inventory, provide additional aid in evaluating and tracking behavioral changes in patients with dementia.[12]

The neurobiology of behavioral manifestations involves a correlation between the decreasing cholinergic function, the depletion of serotonin and norepinephrine levels in depressive and agitation symptoms, and the dysregulation of γ-aminobutyric acid, serotonin, and norepinephrine in association with aggressiveness and impulsivity.[13]

There is currently no Food and Drug Administration (FDA)–approved medication to treat these common and debilitating behavioral problems. Antipsychotic medications have been used off label, but the FDA black-box warning that links these medications to increased mortality (most commonly from cardiac or infectious causes) and research findings that emphasize either modest medication efficacy or lack of it significantly curtail prescribing practices.[14]

DEPRESSION

Out of the various psychiatric disorders in the elderly, depression is most common. However, it is often underdiagnosed and inadequately treated.[15,16] The symptoms

INSTRUCTIONS: Rate the severity of the following symptoms of delirium based on current interaction with subject or assessment of his/her behavior or experience over past several hours (as indicated in each item.)

ITEM 1-REDUCED LEVEL OF CONSCIOUSNESS (AWARENESS): Rate the patient's current awareness of and interaction with the environment (interviewer, other people/objects in the room; for example, ask patients to describe their surroundings).

☐ 0: none   (patient spontaneously fully aware of environment and interacts appropriately)
☐ 1: mild   (patient is unaware of some elements in the environment, or not spontaneously interacting appropriately with the interviewer; becomes fully aware and appropriately interactive when prodded strongly; interview is prolonged but not seriously disrupted)
☐ 2: moderate   (patient is unaware of some or all elements in the environment, or not spontaneously interacting with the interviewer; becomes incompletely aware and inappropriately interactive when prodded strongly; interview is prolonged but not seriously disrupted)
☐ 3: severe   (patient is unaware of all elements in the environment with no spontaneous interaction or awareness of the interviewer, so that the interview is difficult-to-impossible, even with maximal prodding)

ITEM 2-DISORIENTATION: Rate current state by asking the following 10 orientation items: date, month, day, year, season, floor, name of hospital, city, state, and country.

☐ 0: none   (patient knows 9-10 items)
☐ 1: mild   (patient knows 7-8 items)
☐ 2: moderate   (patient knows 5-6 items)
☐ 3: severe   (patient knows no more than 4 items)

ITEM 3-SHORT-TERM MEMORY IMPAIRMENT: Rate current state by using repetition and delayed recall of 3 words [patient must immediately repeat and recall words 5 min later after an intervening task. Use alternate sets of 3 words for successive evaluations (for example, apple, table, tomorrow, sky, cigar, justice)].

☐ 0: none   (all 3 words repeated and recalled)
☐ 1: mild   (all 3 repeated, patient fails to recall 1)
☐ 2: moderate   (all 3 repeated, patient fails to recall 2-3)
☐ 3: severe   (patient fails to repeat 1 or more words)

ITEM 4-IMPAIRED DIGIT SPAN: Rate current performance by asking subjects to repeat first 3, 4, then 5 digits forward and then 3, then 4 backwards; continue to the next step only if patient succeeds at the previous one.

☐ 0: none   (patient can do at least 5 numbers forward and 4 backward)
☐ 1: mild   (patient can do at least 5 numbers forward, 3 backward)
☐ 2: moderate   (patient can do 4-5 numbers forward, cannot do 3 backward)
☐ 3: severe   (patient can do no more than 3 numbers forward)

Fig. 1. MDA scale. (*From* Breitbart W, Rosenfeld B, Roth A, et al. The memorial delirium assessment scale. J Pain Symptom Manage 1997;13(3):128–37; with permission.)

of depression may overlap with various medical disorders. A meta-analysis of 20 prospective studies on depression among elderly subjects indicated that various factors, such as bereavement, sleep disturbance, disability, prior depression, and female sex, were associated with an increased risk for depression.[17] Unrecognized and untreated depression is associated with increased morbidity and mortality from coexisting conditions and suicide.[18]

Depression is the most common risk factor in elderly individuals who commit suicide, reported to be as high as 85%.[19] As compared with younger individuals, it has

ITEM 5-REDUCED ABILITY TO MAINTAIN AND SHIFT ATTENTION: As indicated during the interview by questions needing to be rephrased and/or repeated because patient's attention wanders, patient loses track, patient is distracted by outside stimuli or over-absorbed in a task.

- ☐ 0: none   (none of the above; patient maintains and shifts attention normally)
- ☐ 1: mild   (above attentional problems occur once or twice without prolonging the interview)
- ☐ 2: moderate (above attentional problems occur often, prolonging the interview without seriously disrupting it)
- ☐ 3: severe (above attentional problems occur constantly, disrupting and making the interview difficult-to-impossible)

ITEM 6-DISORGANIZED THINKING: As indicated during the interview by rambling, irrelevant, or incoherent speech, or by tangential, circumstantial, or faulty reasoning. Ask patient a somewhat complex question (for example, "Describe your current medical condition.").

- ☐ 0: none   (patient's speech is coherent and goal-directed)
- ☐ 1: mild   (patient's speech is slightly difficult to follow; responses to questions are slightly off target but not so much as to prolong the interview)
- ☐ 2: moderate (disorganized thoughts or speech are clearly present, such that interview is prolonged but not disrupted)
- ☐ 3: severe (examination is very difficult or impossible due to disorganized thinking or speech)

ITEM 7-PERCEPTUAL DISTURBANCE: Misperceptions, illusions, hallucinations inferred from inappropriate behavior during the interview or admitted by subject, as well as those elicited from nurse/family/chart accounts of the past several hours or of the time since last examination.

- ☐ 0: none   (no misperceptions, illusions, or hallucinations)
- ☐ 1: mild   (misperceptions or illusions related to sleep, fleeting hallucinations on 1-2 occasions without inappropriate behavior)
- ☐ 2: moderate (hallucinations or frequent illusions on several occasions with minimal inappropriate behavior that does not disrupt the interview)
- ☐ 3: severe (frequent or intense illusions or hallucinations with persistent inappropriate behavior that disrupts the interview or interferes with medical care)

ITEM 8-DELUSIONS: Rate delusions inferred from inappropriate behavior during the interview or admitted by the patient, as well as delusions elicited from nurse/family/chart accounts of the past several hours or of the time since the previous examination.

- ☐ 0: none   (no evidence of misinterpretations or delusions)
- ☐ 1: mild   (misinterpretations or suspiciousness without clear delusional ideas or inappropriate behavior)
- ☐ 2: moderate (delusions admitted by the patient or evidenced by his/her behavior that do not or only marginally disrupt the interview or interfere with medical care)
- ☐ 3: severe (persistent and/or intense delusions resulting in inappropriate behavior, disrupting the interview or seriously interfering with medical care)

Fig. 1. (*continued*).

been observed that a greater proportion of the elderly who attempt suicide are actually successful.[20]

In diagnosing depression, it is important to consider the *DSM-IV* criteria for major depressive episode as listed here:

- Depressed mood
- Loss of interest
- Anhedonia
- Anorexia
- Insomnia/hypersomnia
- Decreased concentration
- Wishes to die

ITEM 9-DECREASED OR INCREASED PSYCHOMOTOR ACTIVITY: Rate activity over past several hours, as well as activity during interview, by circling (a) hypoactive, (b) hyperactive, or (c) elements of both present.

☐ 0: none   (normal psychomotor activity)
☐ a b c 1: mild   (hypoactivity is barely noticeable, expressed as slightly slowing of movement. Hyperactivity is barely noticeable or appears as simple restlessness.)
☐ a b c 2: moderate   (hypoactivity is undeniable, with marked reduction in the number of movements or marked slowness of movement; subject rarely spontaneously moves or speaks. Hyperactivity is undeniable, subject moves almost constantly; in both cases, exam is prolonged as a consequence.)
☐ a b c 3: severe   (hypoactivity is severe; patient does not move or speak without prodding or is catatonic. Hyperactivity is severe; patient is constantly moving, overreacts to stimuli, requires surveillance and/or restraint; getting through the exam is difficult or impossible.)

ITEM 10-SLEEP-WAKE CYCLE DISTURBANCE (DISORDER OF AROUSAL): Rate patient's ability to either sleep or stay awake at the appropriate times. Utilize direct observation during the interview, as well as reports from nurses, family, patient, or charts describing sleep-wake cycle disturbance over the past several hours or since last examination. Use observations of the previous night for morning evaluations only.

☐ 0: none   (at night, sleeps well; during the day, has no trouble staying awake)
☐ 1: mild   (mild deviation from appropriate sleepfulness and wakefulness states: at night, difficulty falling asleep or transient night awakenings, needs medication to sleep well; during the day, reports periods of drowsiness or, during the interview, is drowsy but can easily fully awaken him/herself)
☐ 2: moderate   (moderate deviations from appropriate sleepfulness and wakefulness states: at night, repeated and prolonged night awakening; during the day, reports of frequent and prolonged napping or, during the interview, can only be roused to complete wakefulness by strong stimuli)
☐ 3: severe   (severe deviations from appropriate sleepfulness and wakefulness states: at night, sleeplessness; during the day, patient spends most of the time sleeping or, during the interview, cannot be roused to full wakefulness by any stimuli)

Fig. 1. (continued).

Box 3
Possible causes of BPSD

Medication side effects: especially anticholinergic, antimuscarinic

Delirium (infection, dehydration, acute medical illness)

Pain linked to chronic or acute medical problems

Frustration caused by progressive memory/cognitive failure

Physical needs (hunger, need for toileting)

Emotional needs (separation from family)

Environmental overstimulation (noise, overcrowding, understimulation)

Rigid caregiving

From Piechniczek-buczek J. Psychiatric emergencies in the elderly. Psychiatr Times 2010. Available at: http://www.psychiatrictimes.com/special-reports/psychiatric-emergencies-elderly/page/0/1.

- Fatigue
- Psychomotor agitation
- Worthlessness/guilt

Antidepressants are considered safe and effective in targeting depressive symptoms. In elderly patients, selective serotonin reuptake inhibitors (SSRIs) are generally well tolerated and have fewer sedative and anticholinergic adverse effects as well as a reduced risk of lethal overdose compared with tricyclic antidepressants.[19]

Psychotherapeutic interventions that enhance adherence to treatment, provide education, increase self-esteem, strengthen social supports, and diminish hopelessness are clinically recommended.[21] Studies also support the effectiveness of electroconvulsive therapy for treatment of geriatric depression[22]; but adverse effects, such as cardiac complications, cognitive decline, or delirium, limit its use in some patients.

SUICIDE

Among all the age groups, elderly people have the highest risk of death caused by suicide. The risk is much higher among elderly people older than 85 years, whereby the suicide rate has been reported to be higher than 18 per 100,000 individuals.[23] It has been observed that elderly people use more violent methods for attempting suicide, such as shooting with handgun, jumping, and hanging.[24–26] The elderly plan their suicidal act over a period of time compared with younger individuals who often committed it impulsively. As compared with the younger individuals, it has been observed that, in the elderly population, a greater proportion of attempted suicides culminate in a fatal outcome.[20]

Elderly persons with underlying psychiatric illness are at a high risk of attempting suicide. In most of these cases, affective illness has been found to be the primary underlying psychiatric illness in 54% to 87% of cases.[27] A history of substance abuse, particularly alcohol dependence is commonly associated with a risk of completed suicide. Elderly persons with multiple comorbid conditions are at a higher suicide risk. In a study of 1354 elderly patients who died of suicide, various associated chronic medical illnesses were commonly present. Inability to cope up with various stressful life events, which accompany later life, such as bereavement, financial stressor due to retirement, lack of social support and physical disability, are associated with increased suicidal tendencies.[28] Pathways of certain biomarkers such as serotonin, nor-adrenaline and neuro-hormones have been associated with higher suicidal tendencies.[29] Personality traits, such as hopelessness, seclusiveness, hostility, timidity, and a rigid lifestyle, have been noted to be associated with suicidal tendencies in the geriatric population.

Nearly 90% of elderly suicide cases have an underlying major psychiatric illness.[28] Conwell and colleagues[30] reported that more than 70% of the elderly suicide victims had visited their primary care physician within a month before attempting suicide. Of these, nearly a third were seen within a week before the act of suicide.

These findings indicate that detailed evaluation of elderly patients can identify those who are at a higher risk of suicide. All patients must undergo a detailed physical and psychological evaluation. In patients with a high risk of suicide, hospitalization should be advised, as it would also help in exploring the underlying cause of suicidal ideation and any coexisting chronic illnesses and their management. In patients with severe depression, it is imperative to start treatment.

ALCOHOL DEPENDENCE AND SUBSTANCE ABUSE

Alcohol dependence and substance abuse are common problems in the elderly and are frequently overlooked by the ED staff. The prevalence of alcohol dependence in the elderly ranges from 0.6% to 3.7%, and the incidence of heavy drinking (between 12–21 drinks per week) is from 3% to 9%.[31] Although the use of alcohol declines in older age groups, the rates of heavy drinking among elderly persons are much higher as compared with a younger individual. Most elderly individuals with alcoholism are early onset drinkers. On the other hand, a few are late-onset drinkers, who develop problem drinking after a traumatic life event.[32,33] Nearly 0% of elderly men and 10% of elderly women have been reported to have a problem drinking level.[34] Because of impaired metabolism and a decrease in the volume of distribution, alcohol intoxication may occur with a smaller dose of alcohol and withdrawal symptoms may be more pronounced.[35] Factors associated with an increased risk of alcohol abuse in the elderly include social isolation, history of alcohol abuse in the past, and higher educational qualification.[36] In addition, alcohol may interact with various drugs being prescribed for other medical conditions commonly present in the elderly, resulting in adverse effects.

Common presenting symptoms of geriatric alcohol and substance abusers in the ED are dementia, delirium, gait disturbances, hypoglycemia, dehydration, hypothermia, Korsakoff psychosis, head and pelvic trauma. All elderly people presenting in ED should be screened for evidence of alcohol and substance abuse. Usually, older people do not volunteer information about alcohol abuse. Various quick screening tools, such as the CAGE (cut down, annoyed, guilty, eye opener) questionnaire and Short Michigan Alcohol Screening Test–Geriatric Version, are available, which may be used.[37]

POLYPHARMACY

Elderly patients are the highest patient population at risk for polypharmacy, with nearly 100,000 patients being admitted annually through the ED for adverse drug events.[38,39] On average, geriatric patients in the ED receive 4.2 medications per day, with 91% receiving at least one and 13% receiving 8 or more drugs.[40] Given these staggering numbers, it is not hard to believe that nearly 11% of ED visits in patients older than 65 years are caused by adverse drug reactions compared with only 4% in the general population. This finding is primarily related to the fact that the elderly have impaired rates of drug metabolism and excretion, which result in adverse clinical outcomes.[41]

Various antipsychotic drugs may be associated with adverse effects, such as tardive dyskinesia, akathisia, and parkinsonism. Rarely, the use of haloperidol may result in life-threatening complications, such as neuroleptic malignant syndrome (NMS), which may present with hyperthermia, dysautonomia, muscular rigidity, cardiac arrhythmias, and renal failure.[42] It is often difficult to differentiate NMS from serotonin syndrome, which is caused by toxicity caused by SSRIs. **Table 1** differentiates NMS from serotonin syndrome.

Table 1 Serotonin syndrome versus NMS		
	Serotonin Syndrome	**NMS**
Onset	Abrupt	Gradual
Course	Rapidly resolving	Prolonged
Clinical findings	Myoclonus & tremor	Diffuse rigidity
Reflexes	Increased	Decreased
Pupils	Mydriasis	Normal

Furthermore, sudden cessation of SSRIs may result in serotonin discontinuation syndrome, which is associated with insomnia, dizziness, and agitation.[43]

Various tricyclic antidepressants should be used carefully in the elderly because they may result in conduction abnormalities and cardiac dysfunction, especially in patients with underlying coronary artery disease. Lithium is commonly used in patients with affective disorders, such as bipolar mania and depression. It has a narrow therapeutic margin, and older patients are at a greater risk for developing lithium toxicity. Use of concomitant medications, such as nonsteroidal antiinflammatory drugs, furosemide, and lisinopril, may precipitate lithium toxicity resulting in drowsiness, ataxia, and respiratory failure, leading to a fatal outcome. Salt restriction and dehydration may aggravate drug toxicity; hence, adequate replenishment of fluids and electrolytes is crucial for managing these patients in the ED. In severe cases, lithium can be removed from the body by emergency hemodialysis.

Benzodiazepines are frequently prescribed among geriatric patients for sleep and anxiety disorders. Prolonged use of benzodiazepines may result in fatigue, somnolence, and gait disturbances, thereby predisposing them to injuries secondary to an increased fall risk. In severe cases, hallucinations, dementia, drug dependence, aggression, and respiratory depression may occur. In cases with acute toxicity caused by benzodiazepines, flumazenil can be effectively used for reversal of symptoms.

ELDER ABUSE AND NEGLECT

Elder abuse and neglect are being recognized as an emerging area of concern for health care providers across various specialties. There are several definitions for describing elder abuse. However, the key components involve an intentional or neglectful act by the caregiver or trusted person, which may result in harm or threaten the well-being of older persons.[44,45] This abuse may take various forms, such as physical abuse, psychological abuse, caregiver neglect, sexual abuse, and financial exploitation.[46,47] Nearly 10.0% of older adults and 5.6% of older couples experience some form of abuse or neglect every year, and there is an increasing trend in its incidence.[48–52]

Various factors that increase the risk for elder abuse may be associated with the elder person, perpetrator, relationships, and environment. In a systematic review of 49 studies, various risk factors for elder abuse were identified and are summarized in **Table 2**.

The pattern of injuries may point toward elder abuse as the underlying etiologic factor. A study on the elderly people presenting in the ED revealed that victims of severe traumatic elder abuse were more likely to have penetrating injuries.[53] The most

Table 2 Risk factors for elder abuse			
Elderly	**Perpetrator**	**Relationship**	**Environment**
Cognitive impairment	Caregiver burden or stress	Familial discordance	Poor social
Behavioral problems	Psychiatric illness	Conflict	support
Psychiatric illness			
Functional dependency			
Poor physical health			
Frailty			
Low income			
Trauma or past abuse			
Ethnicity			

Data from Friedman LS, Avila S, Tanouye K, et al. A case-control study of severe physical abuse of older adults. J Am Geriatr Soc 2011;59:417–22.

common types were open wounds (56%), internal injuries (24%), and fractures (22%). They were more likely to suffer injuries to the head and trunk. Another study assessing the use of ED by victims of elder abuse found that 15.4% of the visits had physical injuries as their presenting complaint.[54]

The Joint Commission has mandated hospitals for written criteria for identifying all victims of violence, including elder abuse.[55] Suspicion of elder abuse may be made in elderly persons who present with multiple injuries, poor general hygiene, malnutrition, and nonadherence to medical care. Eliciting evidence of elder abuse or mistreatment may be difficult on account of several reasons. The elderly may try to misinform the health care provider on account of fear of being ostracized by the caregiver or being placed in a nursing facility. The elderly should be interviewed in the absence of the caregiver; if the need arises, they should be referred to Adult Protective Services.

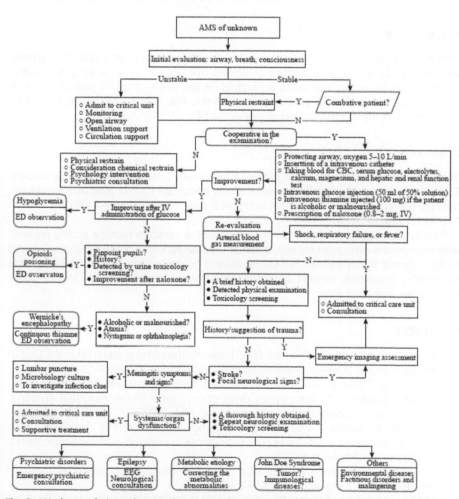

Fig. 2. Work-up of altered mental status in the ED. AMS, altered mental status; CBC, complete blood count; EEG, electroencephalogram; IV, intravenous. (*From* Xiao H, Wang Y, Xu T, et al. Evaluation and treatment of altered mental status in the emergency department: Life in the fast lane. World J Emerg Med 2012;3(4):270–7; with permission.)

Table 3
Differential diagnosis of delirium

	Delirium	Dementia	Depression	Psychotic Illness
Onset	Acute	Gradual	Variable	Variable
Course	Fluctuating	Progressive	Recurrent	Chronic
Consciousness	Altered	Normal	Normal	Normal
Attention	Impaired	Normal until late	May be impaired	May be impaired
Orientation	Fluctuating	Impaired	Normal	Normal
Hallucinations	Common	Rare until late	Rare	Common
Duration	Hours–months	Months–years	Weeks–months	Months–years

From Piechniczek-Buczek J. Psychiatric emergencies in the elderly. Psychiatr Times 2010. Available at: http://www.psychiatrictimes.com/special-reports/psychiatric-emergencies-elderly/page/0/1.

ALTERED MENTAL STATUS

This article would be remiss if it did not include the fact that elderly patients can present to the ED seeming depressed or altered but not for an underlying psychiatric cause. It can be purely related to a medical cause, such as a UTI, sepsis, cerebral hemorrhage, meningitis, or abnormal electrolytes. **Fig. 2** is a concise flow chart on the work-up of the altered mental status in the ED.

SUMMARY

The diagnosis of psychiatric emergencies in the elderly population who presents to the ED is complex and often multifactorial. It is very important the ED clinician differentiate delirium from depression, dementia, and primary psychoses. **Table 3** lists the key differential characteristics.[3,56]

Besides correct diagnosis, it is important that the clinician provide elderly patients with appropriate resources for admission or discharge. Often these resources extend to the patients' family as well; but diagnosis and having a broad differential diagnosis to identify a potentially serious underlying psychiatric emergency in the elderly population is the first, vital step.

REFERENCES

1. Vincent GK, Velkoff VA. The next four decades: the older population in the United States: 2010 to 2050-Grayson K. Vincent, Victoria Averil Velkoff. 2010.
2. Centers for Disease Control and Prevention. National hospital ambulatory medical care survey: 2011 emergency department tables. 2014. Available at: http://www.cdc.gov/nchs/ahcd.htm. Accessed April 24, 2015.
3. Piechniczek-buczek J. Psychiatric emergencies in the elderly. Psychiatr Times 2010. Available at: http://www.psychiatrictimes.com/special-reports/psychiatric-emergencies-elderly/page/0/1.
4. Lipowski ZJ. Transient cognitive disorders (delirium, acute confusional states) in the elderly. Am J Psychiatry 1983;40:1426–36.
5. Fong TG, Tulebaev SR, Inouye SK. Delirium in elderly adults: diagnosis, prevention and treatment. Nat Rev Neurol 2009;5:210–20.
6. Breitbart W, Rosenfeld B, Roth A, Smith MJ, Cohen K, Passik S. The memorial delirium assessment scale. J Pain Symptom Manage 1997;13:128–37.

7. Grover S, Kate N. Assessment scales for delirium: a review. World J Psychiatry 2012;2(4):58–70.
8. American Psychiatric Association. Practice guideline for the treatment of patients with delirium. Arlington (VA): American Psychiatric Publishing Inc; 1999.
9. Overshott R, Karim S, Burns A. Cholinesterase inhibitors for delirium. Cochrane Database Syst Rev 2008;(1):CD005317.
10. Finkel S. Introduction to behavioural and psychological symptoms of dementia (BPSD). Int J Geriatr Psychiatry 2000;15(Suppl 1):S2–4.
11. Aupperle P. Management of aggression, agitation, and psychosis in dementia: focus on atypical antipsychotics. Am J Alzheimers Dis Other Demen 2006;21:101–8.
12. Stoppe G, Brandt CA, Staedt JH. Behavioural problems associated with dementia: the role of newer antipsychotics. Drugs Aging 1999;14:41–54.
13. Tueth MJ. Dementia: diagnosis and emergency behavioral complications. J Emerg Med 1995;13:519–25.
14. Jeste DV, Blazer D, Casey D, et al. ACNP white paper: update on use of antipsychotic drugs in elderly persons with dementia. Neuropsychopharmacology 2008; 33:957–70.
15. Weissman MM, Leaf PJ, Tischler GL, et al. Affective disorders in five United States communities. Psychol Med 1988;18(1):141–53.
16. Meldon SW, Emerman CL, Schubert DS. Recognition of depression in geriatric ED patients by emergency physicians. Ann Emerg Med 1997;30(4):442–7.
17. Cole MG, Dendukuri N. Risk factors for depression among elderly community subjects: a systematic review and meta-analysis. Am J Psychiatry 2003;160(6): 1147–56.
18. Waern M, Runeson BS, Allebeck P, et al. Mental disorder in elderly suicides: a case-control study. Am J Psychiatry 2002;159:450–5.
19. Birrer RB, Vemuri SP. Depression in later life: a diagnostic and therapeutic challenge. Am Fam Physician 2004;69:2375–82.
20. Pearson JL, Brown GK. Suicide prevention in late life: directions for science and practice. Clin Psychol Rev 2000;20(6):685–705.
21. Fiske A, Wetherell JL, Gatz M. Depression in older adults. Annu Rev Clin Psychol 2009;5:363–89.
22. Salzman C, Wong E, Wright BC. Drug and ECT treatment of depression in the elderly, 1996-2001: a literature review. Biol Psychiatry 2002;52:265–84.
23. Conwell Y, Duberstein PR, Cox C, et al. Relationships of age and axis I diagnoses in victims of completed suicide: a psychological autopsy study. Am J Psychiatry 1996;153(8):1001–8.
24. Conwell Y, Rotenberg M, Caine ED. Completed suicides at age 50 and over. J Am Geriatr Soc 1990;38(6):640–4.
25. McIntosh JL, Santos JF. Methods of suicide by age: sex and race differences among the young and the old. Int J Aging Hum Dev 1985–1986;22(2):123–39.
26. Burvill PW. Suicide in the multiethnic population of Australia, 1979-1990. Int Psychogeriatr 1995;7(2):319–33.
27. Szanto K, Mulsant BH, Houck PR, et al. Treatment outcome in suicidal vs. non-suicidal elderly patients. Am J Geriatr Psychiatry 2001;9(3):261–8.
28. Conwell Y, Thompson C. Suicidal behavior in elders. Psychiatr Clin North Am 2008;31(2):333–56.
29. Rifai AH, Reynolds CF, Mann JJ. Biology of elderly suicide. Suicide Life Threat Behav 1992;22(1):48–61.
30. Conwell Y, Olsen K, Caine ED, et al. Suicide in later life: psychological autopsy findings. Int Psychogeriatr 1991;3(1):59–66.

31. Liberto JG, Oslin DW, Ruskin PE. Alcoholism in older persons: a review of the literature. PS 1992;43(10):975–84.
32. Finlayson RE, Hurt RD, Davis LJ Jr, et al. Alcoholism in elderly persons: a study of the psychiatric and psychosocial features of 216 inpatients. Mayo Clin Proc 1988; 63(8):761–8.
33. Hurt RD, Finlayson RE, Morse RM, et al. Alcoholism in elderly persons: medical aspects and prognosis of 216 inpatients. Mayo Clin Proc 1988;63(8):753–6.
34. Fleming MF, Barry KL, Manwell LB, et al. Brief physician advice for problem alcohol drinkers. A randomized controlled trial in community-based primary care practices. JAMA 1997;277(13):1039–45.
35. Morse RM. Substance abuse among the elderly. Bull Menninger Clin 1988;52(3): 259–68.
36. Fink A, Hays RD, Moore AA, et al. Alcohol-related problems in older persons. Determinants, consequences, and screening. Arch Intern Med 1996;156(11):1150–6.
37. Mayfield D, McLeod G, Hall P. The CAGE questionnaire: validation of a new alcoholism instrument. Am J Psychiatry 1974;131:1121–3.
38. Budnitz DS, Lovegrove MC, Shehab N, Richards CL. Emergency hospitalizations for adverse drug events in older Americans. N Engl J Med 2011;365(21): 2002–12.
39. Kim MM, Metlay J, Cohen A, et al. Hospitalization costs associated with warfarin-related bleeding events among older community-dwelling adults. Pharmacoepidemiol Drug Saf 2010;19:731–6.
40. Hohl CM, Dankoff J, Colacone A, et al. Polypharmacy, adverse drug-related events, and potential adverse drug interactions in elderly patients presenting to an emergency department. Ann Emerg Med 2001;38:666–71.
41. Stawicki SP, Kalra S, Jones C, et al. Comorbidity polypharmacy score and its clinical utility: a pragmatic practitioner's perspective. J Emerg Trauma Shock, in press.
42. Center for Disease Control and Prevention, National Center for Injury Prevention and Control. Web based injury statistics query and reposting system [online]. Available at: http://www.cdc.gov/injury/wisqars/. Accessed April 24, 2015.
43. Conwell Y, Duberstein PR. Suicide in elders. Ann N Y Acad Sci 2001;932:132–47.
44. Mills TJ, Talavera F, Harwood R. Diagnostic and treatment guidelines on elder abuse and neglect. Chicago: American Medical Association; 1994. p. 4–24.
45. Hoover RM, Polson M. Detecting elder abuse and neglect: assessment and intervention. Am Fam Physician 2014;89(6):453–60.
46. Kruger RM, Moon CH. Can you spot the signs of elder mistreatment? Postgrad Med 1999;106(2):169–73.
47. National Research Council. Elder mistreatment: abuse, neglect and exploitation in an aging America. Washington, DC: The National Academies Press; 2003.
48. National Center on Elder Abuse at the American Public Human Services Association. The National Elder Abuse Incidence Study. 1998. Available at: http://www.aoa.gov/AoA_Programs/Elder_Rights/Elder_Abuse/docs/ABuseReport_Full.pdf. Accessed May 15, 2015.
49. Dong X, Simon MA. Elder abuse as a risk factor for hospitalization in older persons. JAMA Intern Med 2013;173(10):911–7.
50. Beach SR, Schulz R, Castle NG, Rosen J. Financial exploitation and psychological mistreatment among older adults: differences between African Americans and non-African Americans in a population-based survey. Gerontologist 2010; 50(6):744–57.
51. Acierno R, Hernandez MA, Amstadter AB, et al. Prevalence and correlates of emotional, physical, sexual, and financial abuse and potential neglect in the

United States: the National Elder Mistreatment Study. Am J Public Health 2010; 100(2):292–7.

52. Teaster PB, Dugar T, Mendiondo M, et al. The 2004 survey of adult protective services: abuse of adults 60 years of age and older. Available at: http://www.elderabusecenter.org/pdf/research/apsreport030703.pdf. Accessed April 10, 2015.

53. Friedman LS, Avila S, Tanouye K, et al. A case-control study of severe physical abuse of older adults. J Am Geriatr Soc 2011;59:417–22.

54. Lachs MS, Williams CS, O'Brien S, et al. ED use by older victims of family violence. Ann Emerg Med 1997;30:448–54.

55. Ziminski CE, Phillips LR, Woods DL. Raising the index of suspicion for elder abuse: cognitive impairment, falls, and injury patterns in the emergency department. Geriatr Nurs 2012;33(2):105–12.

56. Farrell KR, Ganzini I. Misdiagnosing delirium as depression in medically ill elderly patients. Ann Intern Med 1995;155:2459–64.

Psychiatric Emergencies in Pregnant Women

Michael P. Wilson, MD, PhD[a,b],*, Kimberly Nordstrom, MD, JD[a,c],
Asim A. Shah, MD[d,e], Gary M. Vilke, MD[a,b]

KEYWORDS

- Emergency psychiatry • Pregnancy • Psychosis • Depression • Bipolar disorder

KEY POINTS

- The management of psychiatric conditions in pregnant women involves a comprehensive evaluation and teamwork.
- Pregnant females presenting with new-onset psychosis are more likely to have a medical cause for illness and require a thorough medical screening and evaluation.
- Routine laboratory testing cannot be recommended for nonpregnant patients with psychiatric disease, but pregnant patients are a special population and may require more testing.
- No psychotropic medications are considered safe in pregnancy, but the risk of not treating may be greater than medications that are not known teratogens.
- Medications like lithium, valproic acid, carbamazepine, and benzodiazepines should generally be avoided if possible.

INTRODUCTION

Mental health-related visits to emergency departments (EDs) are common. From 1992 to 2001, approximately 53 million ED visits in the United States involved a behavioral health emergency.[1] In 2011, approximately 3.9% of visits involved a discharge diagnosis of "mental disorder," although is unknown how many of these visits solely involved pregnant patients.[2]

Although there are increasing numbers of visits to EDs in the United States, clinical research in the field of emergency medicine remains scarce.[3] This gap is especially true

Disclosures: The authors have no financial disclosures relevant to this article.
[a] Department of Emergency Medicine Behavioral Emergencies Research (DEMBER) Lab, San Diego, CA, USA; [b] Department of Emergency Medicine, UCSD Health System, San Diego, CA, USA; [c] Department of Psychiatry, Denver Health Medical Center, University of Colorado School of Medicine, Denver, CO, USA; [d] Department of Psychiatry, Baylor College of Medicine, Houston, TX, USA; [e] Department of Community and Family Medicine, Baylor College of Medicine, Houston, TX, USA
* Corresponding author. Department of Emergency Medicine Behavioral Emergencies Research (DEMBER) Lab, San Diego, CA.
E-mail address: mpwilso1@outlook.com

of research in mental illness in pregnancy, even though pregnancy and the postpartum period have traditionally been thought to be times of increased vulnerability for psychiatric disorders. Despite this, there are few randomized trials in pregnancy. Although community-based studies comparing rates of mental illness in pregnant and nonpregnant females have actually found lower rates of mental illness in pregnant females compared with nonpregnant females, rates of illness, particularly depression, still remain high in this population.[4] Thus, it is likely that emergency physicians will encounter pregnant patients suffering from psychiatric complaints. Despite the lack of clear guidelines, emergency physicians nonetheless play a key role in the treatment of these patients, because failure to diagnose or failure to treat appropriately may lead to serious adverse maternal and fetal outcomes.

MEDICAL SCREENING OF PSYCHIATRIC ILLNESS IN PREGNANCY

The first step in the evaluation of pregnant patients with behavioral disorders in the ED is medical screening to detect medical problems that may be contributory to the ED presentation (Wilson MP, Nordstrom K, Anderson EL, et al. American Association for Emergency Psychiatry Task Force: review and consensus statement on medical assessment of adult psychiatric patients presenting acutely to United States emergency departments. Part II: controversies over medical assessment, and consensus recommendations [indicates reviews of existing literature]. Submitted for publication).[5–7] This process is commonly termed "medical clearance," and is covered more thoroughly elsewhere in this issue.

Defining an Adequate Medical Examination

Several studies have investigated the important elements of emergency medical examinations for psychiatric patients, although no study has specifically evaluated key elements of emergency medical examinations in pregnant patients. There is general consensus that abnormal vital signs are an important first clue to the presence of medical illness. Unfortunately, vital signs outside the normal range can be somewhat misleading in pregnancy.[8] Heart rate, for instance, often increases in pregnant females to compensate for decreasing systemic vascular resistance. Systolic blood pressures also typically decrease in pregnancy, reaching their lowest values around 24 weeks of gestation.[8] Fever, however, may be more useful. Although mild hyperthermia may be common in pregnancy, fever defined as 100.4°F or greater, is more concerning for a medical illness.[9]

Assessment of mental status has also been suggested as an important component of screening patients with psychiatric complaints.[5] Given difficulties in using vital signs, mental status screening may potentially be more important in pregnant, behaviorally disordered patients. Case reports exist in which mental status changes, such as disorientation, were misdiagnosed as new-onset psychosis during a prolonged hospital course for hyperemesis gravidarum.[10] New-onset psychosis is relatively uncommon in pregnancy, but may be seen in rare but life-threatening diseases such as Wernicke's encephalopathy. Although often thought of as a disease of alcohol-using patients, Wernicke's encephalopathy may sometimes be associated with hyperemesis gravidarum.[10,11] Because frank disorientation is relatively uncommon in psychiatric disease, patients with mental status alterations like that of Wernicke's encephalopathy are more likely to have a medical etiology for their symptoms.[12] Although a prospective, randomized trial of the addition of mental status screenings to comprehensive physical examinations has never been performed, studies such as these highlight the importance of a mental status examination in medical screening of psychiatric patients. Expert guidelines, such as those by the American Association for Emergency Psychiatry, also recommend consideration of mental status screening in all patients presenting with psychiatric complaints (Wilson MP, Nordstrom K, Anderson EL, et al. American Association for Emergency Psychiatry Task Force: review and consensus statement on medical assessment of adult psychiatric patients presenting acutely to United States Emergency Departments. Part II: controversies over medical assessment, and consensus recommendations [indicates reviews of existing literature]. Submitted for publication).

The Role of Routine Laboratory and Drug Screen Testing

The role of routine laboratory testing in patients with isolated psychiatric complaints has been controversial in the ED literature. Although early studies such as those by Hall and colleagues[13] have indicated prevalence of medical disease approaching 46% in psychiatric patients, more modern studies have indicated that routine laboratory studies generally add little to the workup, especially if the patient is young with isolated psychiatric complaints.[12,14–16] None of these studies, however, specifically investigated special populations, such as those with new-onset psychiatric illness or patients with pregnancy and, depending on the clinical presentation, more extensive testing may be of greater utility in these populations.

At least 1 study that investigated new-onset psychiatric symptoms found a high proportion of medical illness. Henneman and colleagues[17] investigated 100 consecutive patients aged 16 to 65 years who presented to the ED with new-onset psychiatric complaints and no known past psychiatric history. In this cohort, 63 patients were found to have coexisting medical illness, with history/physical examination alone suggesting disease in only 27 of these 63 patients. The authors concluded subsequently that most adult patients with new-onset psychiatric symptoms have a causative medical illness, and recommended extensive evaluation.

The utility of routine urine drug screens have also been called into question in the ED setting. Studies such as that by Schuckman and colleagues[18] have indicated that self-reporting of illicit drug use is unreliable in the ED; however, several ED studies have indicated that knowledge of a patient's substance use does not often change ED diagnosis or disposition of psychiatric patients.[19–22] Based on studies of this type, the American College of Emergency Physicians stated that routine testing for urine drugs of abuse was unnecessary in the ED.[22] However, this guideline did not concern pregnant patients specifically. In this population, substance use may be important to detect early, because it may have deleterious effects on the fetus and offers an earlier opportunity for counseling and intervention. For this reason, the American College of Obstetrics and Gynecology recommends routinely screening for substance use during prenatal visits.[23] However, the American College of Obstetrics and Gynecology makes no recommendation for ED screening, and does not specifically recommend urine drug screens over screening tools or simply asking the patient about substance use.

AGITATION IN PREGNANCY

An Emergency Nurse Association survey indicated that 54.5% of ED nurses have been physically or verbally abused in the past 7 days.[24] Many of these abuses come from agitated patients. Although most practitioners define agitation as "knowing it when they see it," agitation is more properly defined as an "extreme form of arousal that is associated with increased verbal and motor activity."[12] However, agitation in EDs is surprisingly common, with as many as 1.7 million episodes of agitation annually in

EDs in the United States.[25,26] Most ED care has focused on treatment using restraints and sedation, usually with intramuscular preparations. Although recent literature has criticized this approach as both inhumane and wasteful of ED resources, this approach may be particularly inappropriate for pregnant patients.[27]

Although haloperidol was used in the treatment of hyperemesis gravidarum in earlier decades,[10] there are no well-controlled studies that confirm safety of any antipsychotic or benzodiazepine in pregnancy. Evidence for the safety of antipsychotics other than haloperidol are inconclusive, but depending on medication type, may be associated with increased gestational weight, gestational diabetes, and increased risk of preterm birth.[28] However, because there is no evidence to judge safety in a 1-time dose, as is typically given in the ED, administration guidelines are extrapolated from larger studies of fetal safety.

Benzodiazepines in particular are thought to produce fetal harm, although there is uncertainty about the exact teratogenic effects and the association with ED dosing. The risk of oral cleft in the general population is 6 in 10,000 births, and fetal exposure to benzodiazepines elevates the risk to 7 to 11 in 10,000 births, although these results may be subject to recall bias and confounding factors.[29] Diphenhydramine, which has no proven risk to humans in pregnancy, can be used for its sedative effect, but may be associated with anticholinergic side effects. **Table 1** describes package inserts regarding risks in pregnancy of common ED medications.[30]

Newer literature has called for initial approaches to psychiatric patients using a bundle of measures, not unlike a "resuscitation bundle" in critical care. In this approach, agitated patients are treated initially with verbal deescalation. Although emergency clinicians often perceive themselves as too busy for effective verbal deescalation, thus opting for early use of medication instead, there is some indirect evidence that these techniques may work in nonpregnant patients. In a 2010 study, Isbister and colleagues[31] studied the use of droperidol versus midazolam in Australian EDs, with study investigators being required to attempt verbal deescalation before administering medications. As a result, 60 of 223 security calls (26.9%) were lost to the study after being calmed to the point of no longer needing medication.

Although there are no agreed-upon scripts for verbal deescalation, recent expert guidelines suggest some useful strategies.[32] **Table 2** provides some verbal deescalation strategies. Using these principles, some experts believe that verbal deescalation can often be accomplished in only a few minutes and may allow for the avoidance of medications. This strategy is of particular benefit in pregnant patients, because many medications have contraindications or risks.

Of note, care should be taken while using mechanical restraints in pregnant women, especially during the second and third semesters, to avoid undue pressure on the uterus. Monitoring, to include fetal heart tones and movement, should be done frequently.[33]

Although there are no specific data to guide treatment of agitation in pregnant patients, the following algorithm can be suggested:

- Verbal deescalation as a first-line treatment.
- A comprehensive medical examination to identify the most likely cause of the patient's agitation (ie, medical cause vs recurrence of psychiatric disease).
- Treatment of most likely cause of the agitation.
  - If medications cannot be avoided, use the lowest dose possible of a medication that the patient has taken before, unless this medication is a known teratogen.

Table 1	
Package inserts about pregnancy risks for selected drugs	
Drug Name	**Package Insert [dailymed.nlm.nih]**
Alprazolam	"Benzodiazepines can potentially cause fetal harm when administered to pregnant women. If alprazolam tablets are used during pregnancy, or if the patient becomes pregnant while taking this drug, the patient should be apprised of the potential hazard to the fetus...Because use of these drugs is rarely a matter of urgency, their use during the first trimester should almost always be avoided."
Carbamazepine	"Carbamazepine can cause fetal harm when administered to a pregnant woman."
Diphenhydramine	"Research studies with animals haven't found a risk to unborn babies, but it hasn't been properly studied in humans."
Droperidol	"INAPSINE administered intravenously has been shown to cause a slight increase in mortality of the newborn rat at 4.4 times the upper human dose....There are no adequate and well-controlled studies in pregnant women. INAPSINE should be used during pregnancy only if the potential benefit justifies the potential risk to the fetus."
Haloperidol	"There are no well-controlled studies with haloperidol in pregnant women. There are reports, however, of cases of limb malformations observed following maternal use of haloperidol along with other drugs which have suspected teratogenic potential during the first trimester of pregnancy. Causal relationships were not established in these cases. Since such experience does not exclude the possibility of fetal damage due to haloperidol, this drug should be used during pregnancy or in women likely to become pregnant only if the benefit clearly justifies a potential risk to the fetus."
Lithium	"In humans, lithium carbonate may cause fetal harm when administered to a pregnant woman. Data from lithium birth registries suggest an increase in cardiac and other anomalies, especially Ebstein's anomaly."
Lorazepam	"LORAZEPAM MAY CAUSE FETAL DAMAGE WHEN ADMINISTERED TO PREGNANT WOMEN. Ordinarily, lorazepam injection should not be used during pregnancy except in serious or life-threatening conditions where safer drugs cannot be used or are ineffective."
Olanzapine	"This drug should be used during pregnancy only if the potential benefit justifies the potential risk to the fetus."
Risperidone	"Adequate and well controlled studies with risperidone have not been conducted in pregnant women. Neonates exposed to antipsychotic drugs (including risperidone) during the third trimester of pregnancy are at risk for extrapyramidal and/or withdrawal symptoms following delivery...Risperidone should be used during pregnancy only if the potential benefit justifies the potential risk to the fetus."
Valproic acid	"VALPROATE CAN PRODUCE TERATOGENIC EFFECTS. DATA SUGGEST THAT THERE IS AN INCREASED INCIDENCE OF CONGENITAL MALFORMATIONS ASSOCIATED WITH THE USE OF VALPROATE BY WOMEN WITH SEIZURE DISORDERS DURING PREGNANCY WHEN COMPARED TO THE INCIDENCE IN WOMEN WITH SEIZURE DISORDERS WHO DO NOT USE ANTIEPILEPTIC DRUGS DURING PREGNANCY."
Ziprasidone	"There are no adequate and well-controlled studies in pregnant women. Ziprasidone should be used during pregnancy only if the potential benefit justifies the potential risk to the fetus."

Table 2
Useful verbal strategies in verbal deescalation

Suggested Conversational Prompt	Strategy
"What helps you at times like this?"	Invite the patient's ideas
"I think you would benefit from medication."	Stating a fact
"I really think you need a little medicine."	Persuading
"You're in a terrible crisis. Nothing's working. I'm going to get you some emergency medication. It works well and it's safe. If you have any serious concerns, let me know."	Inducing
"I'm going to have to insist."	Coercing; great danger, last resort.

SPECIFIC DISORDERS DURING PREGNANCY

The incidence and prevalence of anxiety disorders in pregnancy is largely unknown,[34,35] although some disorders are thought to be exacerbated by pregnancy.[36] Anxiety symptoms in the pregnant female can be a serious concern for the mother and the fetus. For the mother, heightened anxiety can cause significant physical as well as emotional distress. Emergent conditions, such as abruption[37] and preterm labor,[38,39] have also been associated with anxiety in the mother, with up to a 4-fold increase of preterm labor in women with posttraumatic stress disorder and a major depressive episode after controlling for medications.[39] Lower Apgar score and birthweight is also a known consequence of severe anxiety.[40]

Obsessive–compulsive disorder is known to worsen with pregnancy and during the antepartum period.[41] When exacerbated, obsessive–compulsive disorder can seem to be very similar to acute psychosis. If symptoms are severe, especially if the symptoms seem to be harming the mother or fetus, hospitalization may be required.

The ED management of patients with severe anxiety is similar to that of agitation. Benzodiazepines, which are first-line medications for anxiety, have known harmful effects on the fetus. Diphenhydramine, although not potentially harmful, may cause anticholinergic side effects and would accomplish little more than sedation. If anxiety is severe, the use of benzodiazepines is determined after considering the risks and benefits of their short-term use. If benzodiazepines are used, the risks and benefits, as well as alternatives must to be clearly discussed with the patient and documented in the chart. If anxiety is moderate, instructing the patient on quick relaxation techniques, such as deep, diaphragmatic breathing might be helpful. Patients who present to the ED with anxiety should be screened for a co-occurring mood disorder, because these patients are at a greater risk for depression as well as suicide.[42]

Mood Disorders During Pregnancy

The average age of onset for most mood disorders tends to coincide with peak child-bearing years.[35,43] Rates of major depressive disorder are higher in females, and perhaps highest in childbearing years, although at least 1 study has found lower rates of depression in pregnant compared with nonpregnant females.[4,44]

Depression may be underdiagnosed in pregnancy, partly owing to overlapping symptoms such as low energy, sleep pattern changes, and alterations in appetite. Unfortunately, a mild depressive episode can rapidly become more severe, leading to decreased functioning for the patient. Studies have repeatedly shown that patients will have some form of contact with a medical provider in the weeks before suicide.[45] One study reported that up to 69% may present to the ED for a non–suicide-related issue before suicide.[46] Making detection more difficult, patients present for somatic complaints and do not offer information on worsening mood or decreased interest and pleasure unless asked. Screening is, therefore, key in the ED setting (See 'DSM-5 Diagnostic Criteria for Major Depressive Disorder' in The diagnostic and statistical manual of mental disorders. American Psychiatric Association. 5th edition. Available at: http://www.dsm5.org/).

Many treatments, in the form of psychotherapy and psychopharmacology, are available for the depressed patient. If the patient has a mild depression, referral to outpatient psychotherapy may be sufficient. As severity progresses, however, the treatment must become more aggressive. This treatment may include medication, although there is controversy as to whether to start an antidepressant in the ED. Sources have suggested that it is only safe to do so when there is adequate and secure follow-up for the patient.[47] Selective serotonin reuptake inhibitors, felt to be relatively safe medications, can cause multiple side effects in the mother. These side effects, along with other factors, may lead to early discontinuation of treatment, which increases risk of problematic outcomes.[48] Also, the initiation of these medications, or serotonin norepinephrine reuptake inhibitors, can themselves cause anxiety. For the anxious patient, it is generally recommended to start at half the normal starting dose for the first 1 to 2 weeks.[47] When a patient has severe depression, especially if having associated psychosis, admission to a psychiatric hospital is necessary. The threshold for admission is generally lower in a pregnant and postpartum patient owing to the high incidence of psychosis and the importance of maternal and fetal well-being.

For the postpartum patient, recognizing depression is necessary to help the patient and baby. Severe depression can cause the mother to not properly care for the infant or may cause psychosis, which can lead to direct harm of the infant. Psychosis may be as frequently as 1 in every 1000 deliveries.[49]

Patients with bipolar I disorder may present to the ED in a manic state. Treatment in this setting will mostly focus on agitation (see "Agitation in Pregnancy"). Atypical antipsychotic medications may be preferred in pregnancy over medications like lithium or valproate, but themselves have a number of side effects (see **Table 1**). If the patient recently and abruptly stopped a medication, the safest course might be to restart this medication, although possible exceptions to this would be if the medication is a known teratogen, especially during early pregnancy. Acutely, treatment is in the form of antipsychotic medications and admission to a psychiatric facility.

Psychotic Disorders During Pregnancy

New-onset psychosis in pregnancy is exceptionally rare, with exacerbation of a primary psychotic illness or mood disorder with relapse being much more common.[10] Patients who present to the ED with new-onset psychosis, therefore, require a full medical evaluation for conditions that may have psychosis as a symptom. If this medical evaluation does not reveal an underlying medical condition, treatment is similar to that discussed. Unlike antidepressants, starting antipsychotics in the ED may reduce long-term morbidity, although discussion with the patient about possible fetal harm is mandatory (Nordstrom[47]; see also **Table 1**). In 2004, a Cochrane review noted that since there are no clinical trials of antipsychotic use during pregnancy, no conclusion can be reached as to their efficacy and safety (Webb and colleagues[50]; see also **Table 1**). Although there are no known "safe" antipsychotics in pregnancy, use of medication is generally considered less harmful to the patient and fetus than severe untreated psychosis.

SUMMARY

The management of psychiatric conditions in pregnant women involves a comprehensive evaluation and a strong teamwork between the emergency physician, the obstetrician, and the psychiatrist. Depending on the stage of pregnancy at the time of presentation, a comprehensive support system for the mother and infant are as essential as the medical management of these patients.

Thorough medical screening and evaluation should take place for all pregnant patients presenting with psychiatric complaints. Physicians should "examine thoroughly and test selectively."[5] There should be consideration for more extensive testing in patients with new-onset psychiatric disease, especially psychosis, because this is less common among pregnant patients. Mental status examinations may be useful in this population to specifically exclude delirium.

There is controversy over the use of routine laboratory testing, and this cannot be recommended for nonpregnant patients with exacerbations of existing psychiatric disease. However, pregnant patients are a special population, and emergency physicians should have a lower threshold to obtain laboratory evaluations in these patients.

Although no psychotropic medications are considered safe in pregnancy, the risk associated with the illness is greater than the known risks of medications, which are not known teratogens. In mild to moderate depression and anxiety, medication can largely be avoided if psychotherapy with close follow-up can be arranged. For severe depression, mania, and psychosis, medication may be necessary. If so, medications like lithium, valproic acid, carbamazepine, and benzodiazepines should generally be avoided.

REFERENCES

1. Larkin GL, Claassen CA, Emond JA, et al. Trends in U.S. emergency department visits for mental health conditions, 1992 to 2001. Psychiatr Serv 2005;56:671–7.
2. National Hospital Ambulatory Medical Care Survey: 2011 emergency department summary tables. Available at: www.cdc.gov/nchs/ahcd.htm. Accessed May 26, 2015.
3. Wilson MP, Vilke GM, Ramanujam P, et al. Emergency physicians research commonly encountered patient-oriented problems in proportion to their frequency. West J Emerg Med 2012;13(4):344–50.
4. Vesga-Lopez O, Blanco C, Keye K, et al. Psychiatric disorders in pregnant and postpartum women in the United States. Arch Gen Psychiatry 2008;65(7): 805–15.
5. Tolia V, Wilson MP. The medical clearance process for psychiatric patients presenting acutely to emergency departments. In: Zun LS, Chepenik LG, Mallory MNS, editors. Behavioral emergencies: a handbook for emergency physicians. Cambridge (United Kingdom): Cambridge University Press; 2013. p. 19–24 (indicates reviews of existing literature).
6. Zun LS. Evidence-based evaluation of psychiatric patients. J Emerg Med 2005; 28(1):35–9 (indicates reviews of existing literature).
7. Szpakowicz M, Herd A. "Medically cleared": how well are patients with psychiatric presentations examined by emergency physicians? J Emerg Med 2008;35(4): 369–72.

8. Carlin A, Alfirevic Z. Physiological changes of pregnancy and monitoring. Clin Obstet Gynecol 2008;22(5):801–23.
9. Edwards MJ. Review: hyperthermia and fever during pregnancy. Birth Defects Res Part A 2006;76(7):506–17.
10. Watkins ME, Newport DJ. Psychosis in pregnancy. Obstet Gynecol 2009;113(6): 1349–53.
11. Chiossi G, Neri I, Cavazzuti M, et al. Hyperemesis gravidarum complicated by Wernicke Encephalopathy: background, case report, and review of the literature. Obstet Gynecol Surv 2006;61(4):255–68.
12. Nordstrom K, Zun LS, Wilson MP, et al. Medical evaluation and triage of the agitated patient: consensus statement of the American Association for Emergency Psychiatry Project BETA Medical Evaluation Workgroup. West J Emerg Med 2012;13(1):3–10 (indicates reviews of existing literature).
13. Hall RCW, Gardner ER, Popkin MK, et al. Unrecognized physical illness prompting psychiatric admission. Am J Psychiatry 1981;138(5):629–35.
14. Janiak BD, Atteberry S. Medical clearance of the psychiatric patient in the emergency department. J Emerg Med 2012;43(5):866–70.
15. Amin M, Wang J. Routine laboratory testing to evaluate for medical illness in psychiatric patients in the emergency department is largely unrevealing. West J Emerg Med 2009;20:97–100.
16. Korn CS, Currier GW, Henderson SO. "Medical clearance" of psychiatric patients without medical complaints in the emergency department. J Emerg Med 2000; 18(2):173–6.
17. Henneman PL, Mendoza R, Lewis RJ. Prospective evaluation of emergency medical department clearance. Ann Emerg Med 1994;24:672–7.
18. Schuckman H, Hazelett S, Powell C, et al. A validation of self-reported substance use with biochemical testing among patients presenting to the emergency department seeking treatment for backache, headache, and toothache. Subst Use Misuse 2008;43(5):589–95.
19. Schiller MJ, Shumway M, Batki SL. Utility of routine drug screening in a psychiatric emergency setting. Psychiatr Serv 2000;51(4):474–8.
20. Fortu JMT, Kim K, Cooper A, et al. Psychiatric patients in the pediatric emergency department undergoing routine urine toxicology screens for medical clearance. Pediatr Emerg Care 2009;25:387–92.
21. Eisen JS, Silvilotti MLA, Boyd KU, et al. Screening urine for drugs of abuse in the emergency department: do test results affect patient care decisions? CJEM 2004;6(2):104–11.
22. Lukens TW, Wolf SJ, Edlow JA, et al, for the American College of Emergency Physicians. Clinical policy: critical issues in the diagnosis and management of the adult psychiatric patient in the emergency department. Ann Emerg Med 2006; 47(1):79–99 (indicates reviews of existing literature).
23. American College of Obstetricians and Gynecologists Committee on Health Care for Underserved Women. ACOG Committee opinion No. 473. Substance abuse reporting and pregnancy: the role of the obstetrician-gynecologist. Obstet Gynecol 2011;117:200–1.
24. Emergency Nurses Association Institute for Nursing Research: emergency department violence surveillance study. August 2010. Available at: https://www.ena.org/practice-research/research/Documents/ENAEDVSReportNovember2011.pdf. Accessed September 2, 2011.

25. Zeller SL, Rhoades RW. Systematic reviews of assessment measures and pharmacologic treatments for agitation. Clin Ther 2010;32:403–25 (indicates reviews of existing literature).

26. Zeller SL, Holloman GH, Wilson MP. Management of agitation. Chapter in section 10, "Emergency psychiatry and violence,". In: Tasman A, Lieberman JA, Kay J, et al, editors. Psychiatry. 4th edition. Oxford (United Kingdom): Wiley Publishing; 2014 (indicates reviews of existing literature).

27. Holloman GH, Zeller SL. Overview of project BETA: best practices in evaluation and treatment of agitation. West J Emerg Med 2012;13(1):1–2.

28. Oyebode F, Rastogi A, Berrisford G, et al. Psychotropics in pregnancy: safety and other considerations. Pharmacol Ther 2012;135:71–7.

29. Yonkers KA, Wisner KL, Stowe Z, et al. Management of bipolar disorder during pregnancy and the postpartum period. Am J Psychiatry 2004;161(4): 608–20.

30. Available at: http://dailymed.nlm.nih.gov/dailymed/drugInfo. Accessed May 30, 2015.

31. Isbister GK, Calver LA, Page CB, et al. Randomized controlled trial of intramuscular droperidol versus midazolam for violence and acute behavioral disturbance: the DORM study. Ann Emerg Med 2010;56:392–401.

32. Richmond JS, Berlin JS, Fishkind A, et al. Verbal de-escalation of the agitated patient: consensus statement of the American association for emergency psychiatry project BETA de-escalation workgroup. West J Emerg Med 2012;13(1):17–25 (indicates reviews of existing literature).

33. Mills MD, Berkowitz P. Psychiatric emergencies in pregnancy. In: Foley MR, Stron TH, Garite TJ, editors. Obstetric intensive care manual. 3rd edition. New York: McGraw Hill Inc; 2011 (indicates reviews of existing literature).

34. Goodman JH, Chenausjy KL, Freeman MP. Anxiety disorders during pregnancy: a systematic review. J Clin Psychiatry 2014;75(10):1153–84 (indicates reviews of existing literature).

35. Anderson E. Management of psychiatric illness in pregnancy in the emergency department. Chapter 35. In: Zun LS, Chepenik LG, Mallory MNS, editors. Behavioral emergencies for the emergency physician. Cambridge University Press; 2013 (indicates reviews of existing literature).

36. Altshuler LL, Hendrick V, Cohen LS. An update on mood and anxiety disorders during pregnancy and the postpartum period. Prim Care Companion J Clin Psychiatry 2000;2:217–22.

37. Cohen LS, Rosenbaum JF, Heller VL. Panic attack-associated placental abruption: a case report. J Clin Psychiatry 1989;50(7):266–7.

38. Dole N, Savitz DA, Hertz-Picciotto I, et al. Maternal stress and preterm birth. Am J Epidemiol 2003;157(1):14–24.

39. Yonkers KA, Smith MV, Forray A, et al. Pregnant women with posttraumatic stress disorder and risk of preterm birth. JAMA Psychiatry 2014;71(8):897–904.

40. Wadhwa PD, Sandman CA, Porto M, et al. The association between prenatal stress and infant birth weight and gestational age at birth: a prospective investigation. Am J Obstet Gynecol 1993;169(4):858–65.

41. Labad J, Menchon JM, Alonso P, et al. Female reproductive cycle and obsessive-compulsive disorder. J Clin Psychiatry 2005;66(4):428–35.

42. Sareen J, Cox BJ, Afifi TO, et al. Anxiety disorders and risk for suicidal ideation and suicide attempts: a population-based longitudinal study of adults. Arch Gen Psychiatry 2005;62:1249–57.

43. Weissman MM, Bland R, Joyce PR, et al. Sex differences in rates of depression: cross-national perspectives. J Affect Disord 1993;29:77–84.
44. Yonkers KA, Vigod S, Ross LE. Diagnosis, pathophysiology, and management of mood disorders in pregnant and postpartum women. Obstet Gynecol 2011; 117(4):961–77 (indicates reviews of existing literature).
45. Wilson MP, Nordstrom K, Zeller SL. Practical management of the suicidal patient in the emergency department. Emerg Med Rep 2014;35(1):1–12 (indicates reviews of existing literature).
46. Gairin J, House A, Owes D. Attendance at the accident and emergency department in the year before suicide: a retrospective study. Br J Psychiatry 2003;183: 28–33.
47. Nordstrom K. Treatment of psychiatric illness in the emergency department. Chapter 27. In: Zun LS, Chepenik LG, Mallory MNS, editors. Behavioral emergencies for the emergency physician. Cambridge University Press; 2013 (indicates reviews of existing literature).
48. Warden D, Madhukar H, Trivedi MD, et al. Early adverse events and attrition in SSRI treatment: a suicide assessment methodology study. J Clin Psychopharmacol 2010;30:259–66.
49. Ohara MW. Post-partum blues, depression and psychosis: a review. J Psychosom Obstet Gynaecol 1987;7(3):205–27.
50. Webb RT, Howard L, Abel KM. Antipsychotic drugs for non-affective psychosis during pregnancy and postpartum. Cochrane Database Syst Rev 2004;(2):CD004411 (indicates reviews of existing literature).

Special Considerations in Trauma Patients

Michael K. Abraham, MD, MS[a],*, Patrick R. Aquino, MD[b], Dick C. Kuo, MD[c]

KEYWORDS

- Traumatic brain injury (TBI) • Chronic traumatic encephalopathy (CTE)
- Trauma evaluation • Posttraumatic stress disorder (PTSD)

KEY POINTS

- Psychiatric patients may present with traumatic injuries that require initial stabilization and trauma resuscitation, and certain situations should warrant direct questioning of suicidality.
- Traumatic brain injury is associated with somatic, cognitive, and neuropsychiatric symptoms; a few studies support their association with psychiatric illness and suicide, but there are few good studies available.
- Patients who are at risk for repetitive traumatic brain injury are at risk for chronic traumatic encephalopathy.
- Posttraumatic stress disorder is common, so screening for past traumatic events and re-experiencing of events should be performed in patients with somatic and psychiatric complaints.

INTRODUCTION

Dealing with patients who present with a behavioral health emergency can be challenging. The evaluation of patients with psychiatric disturbances becomes increasingly complex in the setting of traumatic injury. The sequelae of trauma can be experienced both physically and psychologically. For patients with preexisting psychiatric disease, the traumatic injury, evaluation, and recovery period each have particular difficulties

Disclosures: The authors have no conflicts to disclose.

The article was copyedited by Linda J. Kesselring, MS, ELS, the technical editor/writer in the Department of Emergency Medicine at the University Of Maryland School Of Medicine.

[a] Department of Emergency Medicine, University of Maryland School of Medicine, 110 South Paca Street, 6th Floor Suite 200, Baltimore, MD 21201, USA; [b] Department of Psychiatry and Behavioral Medicine, Lahey Hospital and Medical Center, Tufts University School of Medicine, 41 Mall Road, Burlington, MA 01805, USA; [c] Section of Emergency Medicine, Department of Medicine, Baylor College of Medicine, One Baylor Plaza, Houston, TX 77030, USA

* Corresponding author.

E-mail address: mabraham@umem.org

http://dx.doi.org/10.1016/j.emc.2015.07.011
emed.theclinics.com

requiring adept maneuvering by the emergency medicine provider. The presence of psychiatric colleagues can facilitate the recognition of psychiatric disease and improve management of these patients under difficult circumstances. The authors look to describe the general approach of the emergency medicine provider to patients with traumatic injuries with comorbid psychiatric illness and use several common clinical scenarios to highlight particular challenges to providers.

EVALUATION AND TREATMENT
Initial Stabilization

The premorbid mental health condition of patients is generally not known on initial presentation to emergency providers. Initial procedures for stabilizing patients with a major trauma should be stabilized following standard advanced cardiac life support (ACLS) guidelines, with consideration of limiting morbidity and mortality. Patients who have experienced minor trauma should also have a thorough primary trauma assessment of the airway, breathing, and circulations before moving to any other pressing issues. Although each situation can present individual challenges generally, chronic mental health conditions can be deferred until after the initial stabilization. Acutely agitated patients provides a clinical example whereby adjustments in assessment may be required. Provider safety is paramount during the assessment of the acutely agitated patient. Providers may use standard de-escalation techniques to engage patients in the assessment. When this is not possible, rapid tranquilization may be required with the caveat that this may impair the assessment of the patients' neurologic status. One well-prescribed regimen is haloperidol 5 mg intravenously (IV) and lorazepam 2 mg IV with or without the addition of diphenhydramine 25 mg IV. This regimen does require that patients have an IV established, which can be difficult or dangerous depending on the mental status of patients. Some physicians prefer to use benzodiazepines as a single agent in cases of agitation without psychotic features. The most widely used medication in this scenario is a benzodiazepine. The utilization of benzodiazepines satisfy many of the major criteria for use in an emergent situation in that they are easily administered via multiple routes, can be easily titrated, and have very few significant side effects. Nobay and colleagues[1] compared intramuscular (IM) midazolam (5 mg) with IM lorazepam (2 mg) or IM haloperidol (5 mg). All produced sedation, with midazolam having the fastest onset (18.3 minutes) and shortest duration of action (81.9 minutes). Acutely psychotic patients during the initial stabilization may, because of psychosis or paranoia, refuse to participate in care. Here too, common techniques to engage patients and provide a safe environment can facilitate rapport to allow examination, and ultimately treatment, by the provider. Common nonpharmacologic techniques should be attempted before the administration of medications. Some indications that patients are acutely psychotic are that they can be seen talking to themselves, internally distracted, guarded, fearful, or disorganized in their speech. These indications may be clues to the emergency provider to the presence of an acute exacerbation of psychiatric disease. Quick utilization of medications to deliver rapid tranquilization can facilitate a physical examination or allow for imaging. Regardless of the choice of chemical or physical restraints, it is imperative that the emergency provider remains in control of the situation to protect both the staff and patients.

Secondary Evaluation

After the initial stabilization occurs, a thorough history and physical examination must be performed on these patients. Data suggest that history and physical examination can effectively clear patients who present with altered mental status.[2] Laboratory and imaging studies should only be obtained after the proper examination has directed utilization.[3] If the history and physical examination indicate abnormalities in the vital signs, indications of trauma, or other worrisome details, a more extensive work-up will be necessary. Unexplained abnormalities in the vital signs or physical examination should warrant a more extensive investigation into the cause. Observed signs after a motor vehicle collision may be hypertension, tachycardia, or altered mental status; the physiologic abnormalities may be directly caused by traumatic injuries; however, alternative causes must be entertained. Substance use, especially alcohol, is common in patients presenting with traumatic injury.[4] The relative incidence would support the use of routine evaluation of toxicology or alcohol screens for patients presenting after severe traumatic injury. Alcohol intoxication provides a poignant example for clinical providers because intoxication, rather than a withdrawal state, is most likely at the initial presentation. Alcohol intoxication is usually clinically observed by alterations in the patients' sensorium, speech, gait, and movements or by smell. The presence of alcohol intoxication may alter management and limit further psychoactive drugs or sedating agents because of synergistic effects. This situation poses a difficult treatment conundrum for the emergency provider, as the use of sedatives or antipsychotics can both facilitate the evaluation while at the same time exacerbating the effects of alcohol. Airway compromise as a result of excessive sedation is a real concern and would require immediate measures to protect the airway with a nasal airway or intubation. There is no way to effectively determine, using a physical examination alone, whether patients are expressing symptoms consistent with intoxication or a traumatic brain injury (TBI). Therefore, all clinical decision rules pertaining to brain imaging in trauma have intoxication as an exclusion criteria.

In contrast to acute alcohol intoxication, individuals with chronic alcohol use are at an increased risk of developing alcohol withdrawal, even in the presence of a positive blood alcohol level. Alcohol withdrawal can manifest after the initial assessment is complete and during the secondary assessment, or later in the treatment process, by inpatient providers. Acute alcohol withdrawal is a life-threatening emergency requiring rapid detection and intervention to prevent seizures or further clinical destabilization. Acute alcohol withdrawal is most likely to present in the 48- to 72-hour post-consumption window and can be seen in both the emergency department (ED) or as an inpatient. The initial signs of alcohol withdrawal include vital sign abnormalities, including tachycardia and hyperthermia. Later in the process of withdrawal, patients can have hallucinations and other psychotic manifestations. One can easily see the overlap between traumatic injuries, mental health crises, and substance abuse. The emergency medicine provider must maintain vigilance that any one (or a combination) of these clinical entities is present and be able to address them.

For patients with altered mental status, regardless of cause, the secondary evaluation allows for further investigation to be completed. Direct inquiry into past mental health diagnoses, including treatment of substance use, completes a secondary assessment. This information may provide a basis for further clinical interventions, including maintaining patients' safety during further evaluation. Clinical examples of single-passenger motor vehicle crash, multidrug overdose, or fall from height are scenarios whereby direct inquiry into suicidality would be prudent. Inquiry about suicidality does not increase the risk of suicidality and provides direct clinical support to institute further safety measures during extended evaluation. This information may provide additional impetus to engage psychiatric colleagues in the ongoing management of patients.

Specific Conditions

Delirium

Delirium is an acute cerebral state characterized by disturbed consciousness and cognitive dysfunction occurring in the setting of a physiologic derangement caused by a medical disorder.[5] Referred to as an acute confusional state, change in mental status, encephalopathy, or altered mental status, the signs and symptoms of delirium are frequently overlapping with a spectrum of neuropsychiatric disease: disturbances in arousal caused by cerebral hemorrhage or toxidromes, inattention from frontal network dysfunction or hallucinatory experiences, memory disturbance from concussion, or dementia. For patients presenting with traumatic injury, direct acute brain injury should be the prime consideration for the observation of neuropsychiatric symptoms. There is a high incidence of acute confusion in patients with a brain injury.[6] Head imaging, generally brain computed tomography, is warranted to assess intracranial injuries. Rapid sequence intubation may be required to assist in the completion of the necessary evaluation as it can be difficult to ascertain if patients are injured, intoxicated, or psychotic either alone or in some combination of these entities. A detailed neurologic examination including the physical examination of the cranial nerves, reflexes, and strength may localize injuries to guide further work-up. Depending on the necessity of rapid sequence intubation, the neurologic evaluation should occur before paralytics being administered. If paralytics are necessary, the use of short-acting agents like succinylcholine could provide earlier return to neuromuscular baseline and facilitate evaluation. Evaluation with the Glasgow Coma Scale can assist in prognosis as well as provide a measure of serial evaluations. Brief interventions to assess for the presence of delirium have been established in medical and surgical patients, including the confusion assessment method (CAM).[7] The CAM adapted for the intensive care unit setting is designed to be performed in patients who are unable to speak and may be useful as a screening or assessment tool for the emergency provider. Rapid identification of delirium allows the provider to begin a thorough investigation into the cause and, therefore, more rapid correction of the underlying dysfunction.

Traumatic Brain Injury

One of the more common complaints that emergency providers will encounter that crosses into the realm of behavioral health emergencies is TBI. There is a wide spectrum of diseases that encompass the term TBI. Approximately 1% to 2% of ED visits will be attributed to TBIs.[8] Minor TBI (mTBI) can include minor injuries with short recovery time, a mild concussion, and long-term structural brain changes.[9] mTBI can be further subclassified into those with and without loss of consciousness. The incidence of mTBI is estimated at 100 to 300 per 100,000.[10]

TBI has long been associated with neuropsychiatric symptoms as well as somatic symptoms. These neuropsychiatric symptoms are frequently divided into cognitive and behavioral symptoms. Cognitive symptoms include deficits in attention, executive function, and memory. Behavioral symptoms include primary psychiatric disorders, such as mood disorders, psychosis, anxiety, as well as personality disorders. In addition, there are a multitude of somatic complaints associated with TBI that include headache, dizziness, vertigo, seizures, sensitivity to light or sound, hearing loss, and sleep disturbance.[11] There is a decent amount of data that even mTBI is associated with higher rates of neuropsychiatric disorders in both adults and children. In the 6 to 12 months after initial mTBI, patients have higher rates of posttraumatic stress disorder (PTSD), generalized anxiety disorder, and agoraphobia.[12]

TBI not only has short-term effects but can also have effects on long-term outcomes. Studies have also shown that any TBI, even those described as mild, can increase the risk of premature or traumatic death. One study followed subjects in Finland for 15 years after TBI. The subjects had an increased risk of all-cause mortality as well as intentional or unintentional traumatic death.[13] Single-incident TBI is considered a risk factor for Alzheimer disease; according to studies, approximately 20% to 30 % of patients with Alzheimer disease have had a mild to severe TBI at some point in their life.[14] Fann and colleagues[15] showed a significant association with both mild and moderate to severe TBI and psychiatric illness at the 6-month follow-up. They also showed that psychiatric illness was a strong predictor of TBI in their patient population. There are also contradictory studies that claim that head injuries have no bearing on the incidence of schizophrenia in male patients.[16]

It is important to note that the *Diagnostic and Statistical Manual of Mental Disorders* (Fifth Edition) (*DSM-5*) takes a new approach to the diagnosis of TBI and its neuropsychiatric sequelae.[17] The primary focus of *DSM-5* is neurocognitive disorders. The framework for the retrospective diagnosis of TBI is established, and the neurocognitive disorder can be classified as mild or major. The distinctions between the initial severity of TBI is less important, instead focusing on the severity of posttraumatic cognitive deficits and their toll on day-to-day functions.

Neurobehavioral symptoms are reported in almost all patients with TBI in the acute phase after injury,[18] and an estimated 30% to 80% of patients with TBI will have neurobehavioral symptoms for up to 3 months.[19] Various definitions have been used and studies evaluate many different populations, so it is easy to see why the reported incidence varies so widely. The risk factors associated with the development of neurobehavioral symptoms include age, female sex, pain, and prior anxiety or affective disorders.[11,20] Neurobehavioral symptoms persist beyond 3 months in approximately 15% of patients and may contribute to continued societal difficulties.[11,21–23]

Although there is evidence to suggest the association of various neurobehavioral outcomes with TBI, a recent systematic review from the International Collaboration on Mild Traumatic Brain Injury Prognosis concluded that early cognitive effects are common and that recovery may be prolonged.[24] They also reported that a small number of studies indicate that mTBI increases the risk of psychiatric illness and suicide. However, they also noted a great deal of heterogeneity and a lack of well-designed studies to understand the medium-and long-term effects of mTBI.

Other systematic reviews performed by the same group concluded there is a lack of evidence for increased risk of dementia after mTBI[25] and that in children common post-mTBI symptoms and deficits are not specific to mTBI and seem to resolve with time and there is limited evidence that suggests children with intracranial pathology on imaging or complicated TBI may experience persisting symptoms or deficits.[26] Again, well-designed studies are recommended.

Although it is not in the purview of emergency medicine to prevent or typically treat these complications, it is probably worthwhile to ensure that discharge instructions address these issues. Patients with any TBI should have close primary care follow-up and consideration for psychiatric consultation if high recidivism is noted.

CHRONIC TRAUMATIC ENCEPHALOPATHY

Repetitive mTBI may preclude certain individuals to chronic traumatic encephalopathy (CTE). This disease entity has received a great deal of notoriety lately as professional sports teams and military personnel have become increasingly diagnosed with this entity. In 1928, Martland[27] introduced the term *punch drunk*, thus initiating the concept of

CTE. He describes a symptom complex that seemed to be the result of repeated concussive blows to the head. Millspaugh[28] then coined the term *dementia pugilistica* (DP), as this syndrome had long been recognized in professional boxers.[29] Although DP and CTE are classified as separate entities, there is a significant similarity in their presentations.[14] There is a great deal of debate as to the association of CTE and behavioral health issues because there is a tremendous amount of overlap between CTE and other neuropsychiatric diseases. It is also important to note that several of the degenerative tauopathies, one example being variant frontotemporal dementia, have very similar clinicopathologic features of CTE.[30] The comparison of CTE and DP seems to hinge on the age of presentation, with DP presenting much later in life.[14] One common and often overlooked patient population at risk for this entity could be chronic alcoholics who encounter TBI from frequent falls caused by intoxication.

Common presenting symptoms can include memory loss, outbursts of aggressive or violent behavior, confusion, and speech abnormalities, which are not uncommon findings in psychiatric patients in the emergency setting.[29] One retired National Football League football player who had premortem symptoms of a mood disorder consistent with bipolar disease was found to have signs of CTE on autopsy.[31] CTE can have a profound effect on life expectancy, and many patients with CTE do not die of conditions relating to chronic diseases like hypertension or diabetes. An estimated 65% to 80 % of patients die of causes that can include suicide, sequelae from chronic substance abuse, or accidents from irrational and erratic behavior.[14]

The full discussion of diagnosis and current controversies concerning CTE is outside of the realm of this article; however, emergency providers should be aware of the disease and should actively screen patients who are at risk for it. Patients who have experienced repetitive TBI can be at risk for this disease, and the presentation can be solely for behavioral health issues. Currently, emergency providers will not be expected to make the diagnosis of CTE as it can only be made by performing an autopsy, but they should be aware that patients could be at risk for this disease in the proper settings. Future studies will need to be performed to determine if a lumbar puncture can be used to guide the diagnosis of this disease. After medical clearance of these patients from the trauma setting, appropriate referral to psychiatry or neurology for the neuropsychological testing is recommended.

ACUTE STRESS DISORDER AND POSTTRAUMATIC STRESS DISORDER

Injuries from traumatic incidents can extend beyond physical manifestations to psychological injuries. The *DSM-5* identifies a spectrum of traumatic disorders, including adjustment disorders, acute stress disorder, and PTSD.[5] Adjustment disorders are a heterogeneous array of stress-response syndromes that occur after exposure to a distressing (traumatic or nontraumatic) event and interfere with patient functioning in various life domains.

Acute stress disorder and PTSD define a spectrum of psychiatric syndromes that develop after an explicitly defined traumatic event with a constellation of 4 symptom clusters including re-experiencing the event, alterations in arousal, negative experience of cognition, or mood and reactivity. PTSD can be differentiated from other disorders by the re-experiencing of symptoms (ie, nightmares or flashbacks).[32] As discussed earlier, both previous trauma and psychiatric diseases are predictors for subsequent trauma. For individuals with stress disorders, subsequent traumatic events may cause re-experiencing, fear, emotional liability, or withdrawal, all complicating the evaluation and management of patients in the emergency setting. Acutely, it is difficult to determine if patients have experienced a new injury or are presenting with signs of PTSD. Delayed presentations of PTSD are reported in the literature, with one systematic review reporting 25% with delayed PTSD.[33]

PTSD is common, so screening for a history of traumatic events may help solidify the diagnosis. PTSD often present with headaches, sleep disturbances, and pain and may present with depression, substance use, and self-harm. Suicidal behaviors are associated with PTSD.[34]

Standard treatment regimens should be used to safely calm agitated or aggressive patients, including medications like benzodiazepines or antipsychotics. Patients may also experience PTSD from previous medical treatment, including forcible restraints or painful procedures or injuries. Pain seems to be strongly associated with PTSD, and measures to reduce pain have been shown to lower the likelihood of PTSD.[32,35] Thus, it is imperative to consider all of your treatment options in agitated patients, and use the least restrictive measures that ensure safety and to treat pain in an aggressive manner.

In some cases, after a significant traumatic injury has been ruled out, oral medications may be the most effective treatment option. Although their time of onset may be longer when compared with IV or IM medication, the benefits of de-escalation may make the remainder of the treatment more tolerable for patients and staff.

Pharmacotherapy for PTSD includes selective serotonin reuptake inhibitors, such as fluoxetine, sertraline, and paroxetine, and serotonin norepinephrine reuptake inhibitors, such as venlafaxine. These medications have demonstrated efficacy in reducing PTSD symptoms and are considered first-line medication treatments for PTSD.[36,37] However, other medications might be necessary to treat insomnia and nightmares as antidepressants alone are not usually effective.[37] Chronic treatment of PTSD is beyond the scope of this article, although emergency physicians should be familiar with potential medications that patients with PTSD may be taking. In any emergent situation, attending to the patients' needs, providing a safe environment, and addressing any comorbid medical or psychiatric conditions should be the guiding principles of treatment.

SUMMARY

The evaluation for traumatic injuries should include consideration for a behavioral health emergency and vice versa. Patients with behavioral health issues may pose a significant conundrum for the emergency provider, as the trauma may be self-induced or concealed from the provider. Patients who present with behavioral health complaints should receive a thorough medical examination that ensures there are no traumatic injuries. Owing to the overlapping presentations for traumatic injuries and behavioral health emergencies, the emergency provider must maintain an open mind as to the possible cause for the patients' presentation. Although the medical treatment of these patients can be very simple, the complexities inherent in the treatment and long-term outcomes should warrant early consideration for psychiatric consultation or referral.

REFERENCES

1. Nobay F, Simon BC, Levitt MA, et al. A prospective, double-blind, randomized trial of midazolam versus haloperidol versus lorazepam in the chemical restraint of violent and severely agitated patients. Acad Emerg Med 2004;11(7):744-9.
2. Janiak BD, Atteberry S. Medical clearance of the psychiatric patient in the emergency department. J Emerg Med 2012;43(5):866-70.

3. Kanich W, Brady WJ, Huff JS, et al. Altered mental status: evaluation and etiology in the ED. Am J Emerg Med 2002;20(7):613–7.

4. Rivara FP, Jurkovich GJ, Gurney JG, et al. The magnitude of acute and chronic alcohol abuse in trauma patients. Arch Surg 1993;128(8):907–13.

5. American Psychiatric Association. Diagnostic and statistical manual of mental disorders. 5th edition. Washington, DC: American Psychiatric Association Publishing; 2013.

6. Gion T, Leclaire-Thoma A. Delirium in the brain-injured patient. Rehabil Nurs 2014;39(5):232–9.

7. Inouye SK, Van Dyck CH, Alessi CA, et al. Clarifying confusion: the confusion assessment method: a new method for detection of delirium. Ann Intern Med 1990;113(12):941–8.

8. Nakase-Thompson R, Sherer M, Yablon SA, et al. Acute confusion following traumatic brain injury. Brain Inj 2004;18(2):131–42.

9. Iverson GL, Lange RT. Mild traumatic brain injury. In: Schoenberg MR, Scott JG, editors. The little black book of neuropsychology. New York: Springer; 2011. p. 697–719.

10. Vos PE, Alekseenko Y, Battistin L, et al. Mild traumatic brain injury. Eur J Neurol 2012;19(2):191–8.

11. Riggio S, Wong M. Neurobehavioral sequelae of traumatic brain injury. Mt Sinai J Med 2009;76(2):163–72.

12. Gibson R, Purdy SC. Mental health disorders after traumatic brain injury in a New Zealand caseload. Brain Inj 2015;29(3):306–12. Available at: http://search.ebscohost.com/login.aspx?direct=true&db=aph&AN=100928249&site=ehost-live.

13. Vaaramo K, Puljula J, Tetri s, et al. Head trauma with or without mild brain injury increases the risk of future traumatic death: a controlled prospective 15-year follow-up study. J Neurotrauma 2015;32(16):1272–80.

14. Levin B, Bhardwaj A. Chronic traumatic encephalopathy: a critical appraisal. Neurocrit Care 2014;20(2):334–44.

15. Fann JR, Burington B, Leonetti A, et al. Psychiatric illness following traumatic brain injury in an adult health maintenance organization population. Arch Gen Psychiatry 2004;61(1):53–61.

16. Nielsen AS, Mortensen PB, O'Callaghan E, et al. Is head injury a risk factor for schizophrenia? Schizophr Res 2002;55(1):93–8.

17. Wortzel HS, Arciniegas DB. The DSM-5 approach to the evaluation of traumatic brain injury and its neuropsychiatric sequelae. NeuroRehabilitation 2014;34(4):613–23.

18. Lundin A, de Boussard C, Edman G, et al. Symptoms and disability until 3 months after mild TBI. Brain Inj 2006;20:799–806.

19. Rimel RW, Giordani B, Barth JT, et al. Disability caused by minor head injury. Neurosurgery 1981;9:221–8.

20. Meares S, Shores EA, Taylor AJ, et al. Mild traumatic brain injury does not predict acute postconcussion syndrome. J Neurol Neurosurg Psychiatry 2008;79:300–6.

21. Alves W, Macciocchi S, Barth J. Postconcussive symptoms after uncomplicated mild head injury. J Head Trauma Rehabil 1993;8:48–59.

22. Ponsford J, Willmott C, Rothwell A. Impact of early intervention on outcome following mild head injury in adults. J Neurol Neurosurg Psychiatry 2002;73:330–2.

23. Ruff RM, Camenzuli L, Mueller J. Miserable minority: emotional risk factors that influence the outcome of a mild traumatic brain injury. Brain Inj 1996;8:61–5.

24. Carroll LJ, Cassidy JD, Cancelliere C, et al. Systematic review of the prognosis after mild traumatic brain injury in adults: cognitive, psychiatric, and mortality

outcomes: results of the International Collaboration on Mild Traumatic Brain Injury Prognosis. Arch Phys Med Rehabil 2014;95(Suppl 3):S152–73.

25. Godbolt AK, Cancelliere C, Hincapié CA, et al. Systematic review of the risk of dementia and chronic cognitive impairment after mild traumatic brain injury: results of the International Collaboration on Mild Traumatic Brain Injury Prognosis. Arch Phys Med Rehabil 2014;95(Suppl 3):S245–56.

26. Hung R, Carroll LJ, Cancelliere C, et al. Systematic review of the clinical course, natural history, and prognosis for pediatric mild traumatic brain injury: results of the International Collaboration on Mild Traumatic Brain Injury Prognosis. Arch Phys Med Rehabil 2014;95(Suppl 3):S174–91.

27. Martland HS. Punch drunk. J Am Med Assoc 1928;91:1103–7.

28. Millspaugh J. Dementia pugilistica. US Naval Med Bull 1937;35:297–303.

29. McKee AC, Cantu RC, Nowinski CJ, et al. Chronic traumatic encephalopathy in athletes: progressive tauopathy following repetitive head injury. J Neuropathol Exp Neurol 2009;68(7):709–35.

30. McCrory P, Meeuwisse WH, Kutcher JS, et al. What is the evidence for chronic concussion-related changes in retired athletes: behavioural, pathological and clinical outcomes? Br J Sports Med 2013;47(5):327–30.

31. Omalu BI, DeKosky ST, Minster RL, et al. Chronic traumatic encephalopathy in a national football league player. Neurosurgery 2005;57(1):128–34. Available at: http://journals.lww.com/neurosurgery/Fulltext/2005/07000/Chronic_Traumatic_Encephalopathy_in_a_National.21.aspx.

32. Sareen J. Posttraumatic stress disorder in adults: impact, comorbidity, risk factors, and treatment. Can J Psychiatry 2014;59(9):460–7.

33. Smid GE, Mooren TT, van der Mast RC, et al. Delayed posttraumatic stress disorder: systematic review, meta-analysis, and meta-regression analysis of prospective studies. J Clin Psychiatry 2009;70(11):1572–82.

34. Wilcox HC, Storr CL, Breslau N. Posttraumatic stress disorder and suicide attempts in a community sample of urban American young adults. Arch Gen Psychiatry 2009;66(3):305–11.

35. Holbrook TL, Galarneau MR, Dye JL, et al. Morphine use after combat injury in Iraq and post-traumatic stress disorder. N Engl J Med 2010;362(2):110–7.

36. Stein DJ, Seedat S, van der Linden GJ, et al. Selective serotonin reuptake inhibitors in the treatment of post-traumatic stress disorder: a meta-analysis of randomized controlled trials. Int Clin Psychopharmacol 2000;15(Suppl 2):S31–9.

37. Stein DJ, Ipser JC, Seedat S. Pharmacotherapy for post traumatic stress disorder (PTSD). Cochrane Database Syst Rev 2006;(1):CD002795.

Ethical Issues in Emergency Psychiatry

Nathan Gold Allen, MD[a],*, Jeffrey Steven Khan, MD[b],
Mohammad Shami Alzahri, MD, MSc[c,d], Andrea Gail Stolar, MD[b]

KEYWORDS

- Ethics • Decision-making capacity • Confidentiality • Involuntary treatment
- Emergency psychiatry

KEY POINTS

- The capacity of patients with psychiatric illness should be assessed by determining their ability to communicate a choice, understand the relevant information, appreciate the risks and benefits as they apply to them, and rationally manipulate information.
- The need to deliver effective treatment, maintain patient and staff safety, and comply with the law should be balanced against a strong ethical imperative to maintain the confidentiality of psychiatric patients.
- When using involuntary treatment use the least restrictive means possible to achieve the goal of restoring the patient's autonomy, protecting against dangerousness, and addressing impairment from psychiatric illness.

INTRODUCTION

Care of patients with acute psychiatric conditions presents numerous clinical challenges to emergency physicians, including assessment of risk for harm to self and others, assessment of impairment to the patient's decision-making capacity, assessment of the need for hospitalization, evaluation for the presence of an underlying medical condition, the provision of care in an environment of shrinking outpatient and community resources, and the unfortunate but frequent overlap between psychiatric conditions and unstable social situations, substance abuse, and the criminal justice

Financial disclosures: The authors have nothing to disclose.
[a] Section of Emergency Medicine, Department of Medicine, Center for Medical Ethics & Health Policy, Baylor College of Medicine, One Baylor Plaza, Suite 310D, Houston, TX 77030, USA; [b] Menninger Department of Psychiatry and Behavioral Sciences, Baylor College of Medicine, One Baylor Plaza, BCM350, Houston, TX, 77030, USA; [c] Section of Emergency Medicine, Center for Medical Ethics & Health Policy, Baylor College of Medicine, One Baylor Plaza, Houston, TX 77030, USA; [d] King Saud University, Riyadh 12372, Saudi Arabia
* Corresponding author.
E-mail address: Nathan.Allen@bcm.edu

Emerg Med Clin N Am 33 (2015) 863–874
http://dx.doi.org/10.1016/j.emc.2015.07.012
0733-8627/15/$ – see front matter © 2015 Elsevier Inc. All rights reserved.

system. Ethical issues abound in these clinical challenges, and this article enumerates some of the most significant and pressing of them. The broad ethical issues of capacity and consent, confidentiality and privacy, and involuntary treatment are core issues that practicing emergency physicians are likely to confront regularly in the care of patients with emergency psychiatric conditions and, as such, should be prepared to respond to effectively. Although resource use for psychiatric care and failings in the social safety net are important issues, they are not actionable for individual practicing clinicians in the same manner and are not explicitly treated in this article. There are many approaches to analyzing ethical challenges. This article draws most heavily on the work of Beauchamp and Childress[1] and their analysis of ethical issues in terms of autonomy, beneficence, nonmaleficence, and justice.

CAPACITY AND CONSENT

Respect for patients' autonomy is operationalized through the process of informed consent and by allowing patients the right to accept or to refuse medical treatment. However, the ability of individuals to exercise their autonomy can be impaired by various disease states. In such cases, an assessment of a patient's capacity to make the relevant medical decision is warranted. Capacity refers to an individual's ability to make rational decisions, the assessment of which can be completed by health care professionals.[2] Studies show that up to 30% to 50% of patients undergoing a psychiatric admission lack capacity.[3] In addition, in a study of capacity among medical inpatients, clinicians and relatives of the patients rarely detected the presence of incapacity.[4] The prevalence of incapacity and difficulty recognizing it underscore the importance of being able to assess capacity effectively in the emergency department (ED). Any physician can assess capacity, and in the emergency setting all physicians should be prepared to do so. Although a psychiatrist is often helpful in this determination, a psychiatrist is not required to determine a patient's capacity to make medical decisions. Providers should be aware of the inherent bias of only questioning a patient's capacity when the patient is refusing treatment. Even when a patient agrees to treatment, if there is a concern for the patient's ability to make reasoned choices, an assessment is warranted.

Capacity is not an all-or-none phenomenon. Although a patient may retain the ability to decide whether or not to consent to a blood draw, if the risk is low and the benefits potentially high, the patient may not have the ability to rationally weigh the risks, benefits, and alternatives in order to consent to a highly invasive surgical procedure. Thus, the level of capacity required in any particular circumstance increases as the stakes become more significant. Capacity is therefore also situation specific, which means that capacity generally exists on a continuum but is a threshold concept for any specific decision.[5]

Assessing Capacity

When determining capacity, 4 abilities should be assessed, as outlined by Appelbaum and Grisso[6]: the ability to communicate a choice, the ability to understand the relevant information, the ability to appreciate the risks and benefits, and the ability to rationally manipulate the information at hand[6,7] (**Table 1**).

There are tools to assist clinicians in determining decision-making capacity. The MacArthur Competence Assessment Tool for Treatment (MacCAT-T) is one such instrument, and is a validated and reliable tool often used in research.[8] However, emergency physicians may find it easier to use a simpler tool, such as the mnemonic CURVES, developed by clinicians from Johns Hopkins. The first 4 letters correspond

Table 1
Assessing decision-making capacity

Ability	Issue When Absent	Example and Assessment
Communicate a choice	Individuals are unable to express a choice and/or to communicate that choice consistently over time	Patients who are unconscious, incapacitated, or altered. Assessed by asking patients to state a treatment choice
Understand relevant information	Individuals are unable to understand their condition, purpose of treatment, benefits and harms of treatment, alternatives	Patients who have deficits in attention span, intelligence, and memory. Assessed by having patients restate, summarize, or paraphrase information communicated to them
Appreciate the situation and its consequences	Individuals are unable to comprehend that the information provided applies to them or acknowledge likely consequences of their condition	Patients who have deficits in intelligence or understanding, or who have a mental disorder. Assessed by asking questions like, "What might happen to you if you refuse this treatment?" or "Why is this treatment being recommended for you?"
Ability to rationally manipulate information	The individual is unable to use a rational thought process to reach a decision. Note: the process can be rational even if the decision is unreasonable to an external evaluator	Patients who have deficits in intelligence or cognition, or who have a mental disorder that impairs their rational thought processes. Assessed by asking questions like, "Can you help me understand why you are making that choice?" or "What makes that option preferable to you rather than the alternative?"

with the concepts outlined in **Table 1**: choose and communicate, understanding, reason, and value. The last 2 letters E and s (emergency and surrogate) are prompts for the alternative appropriate decision-making strategies to consider when patients lack capacity.[9]

Managing Psychiatric Patients with Uncertain Capacity

Incapacity may be a fluid state and attempts should be made to restore and reassess capacity whenever possible. For example, consider a 40-year-old man with an alcohol use disorder who presents with chest pain, requiring admission for further cardiac evaluation. The patient initially agrees to admission but while boarding in the emergency room becomes frustrated and states a desire to leave against medical advice (AMA). In this case, the reasons for this decision should be reviewed. Such exploration may find that inadequate coverage of alcohol withdrawal symptoms is adversely affecting his thinking. Symptomatic relief could improve his mental status, comfort, and likelihood of complying with medical recommendations, and could preserve his ability to remain capacitated to make medical decisions. Each intervention must be considered in a stepwise fashion, balancing the risks and benefits of the intervention against the risk of inaction in the context of the patient's ability to rationally weigh choices.

Typically, when patients are found to be incapacitated, medical decision making proceeds through either an emergency exception to informed consent or through a surrogate decision maker. This process is not uniformly applicable in emergency psychiatry because, depending on state laws, surrogate decision makers may not be able to consent to voluntary admission or certain treatments. Most states do have laws in place authorizing some type of psychiatric advance directives.[10] These advance directives are similar to other advance directives in that they outline patient care preferences in a similar manner to other advance directives except they are specific for mental health care, such as medication preferences, preferences regarding emergency hospitalization, or preference for use of one form of treatment (medication, restraint, seclusion) rather than another in an emergency. Emergency providers should be aware of and inquire about these directives because they may contain useful information that will help facilitate care for the patient.

Patients with psychiatric illness are significantly more likely to leave the hospital AMA, ranging from 3% to 51% in various studies and averaging 17%.[11] Alcohol (odds ratio [OR], 3.82; 95% confidence interval [CI], 3.56–4.11) and drug abuse (OR, 2.19; 95% CI, 1.99–2.42) are also correlated with risk of leaving AMA, and patients with psychiatric disorders are significantly more likely to have concomitant substance abuse problems as well.[12–14] Aware of these risk factors, emergency physicians should be prepared to respond to patients with primary or coexisting psychiatric illness who are threatening to leave AMA. Further legal and ethical issues to consider in this situation are the balance between patient autonomy and prevention of harm, the availability of alternative treatments, planning for subsequent care, and documentation of the patient encounter. In these situations it is important to consider harms broadly, including both medical harms and harms associated with preventing a patient from leaving. One approach to the challenge of balancing these potentially competing forces is the AIMED (assess, investigate, mitigate, explain, document) strategy proposed by Clark and colleagues[15] and adapted in **Table 2**.

PRIVACY AND CONFIDENTIALITY

Respect for patient privacy and confidentiality is a professional responsibility with both ancient origins and contemporary significance. In the ethics literature a debate remains about whether or not confidentiality is an absolute right in which the harms caused by breaches of confidentiality are never proportional with the potential benefits of violating it, and the argument that choosing to break patient confidentiality is allowable in certain circumstances, such as when required by law, because failure to do so would represent an act of civil disobedience.[16,17] The American College of Emergency Medicine *Principles of Ethics for Emergency Physicians*, in a manner similar to other professional societies, acknowledges this tension and advocates a middle ground, "Emergency physicians shall respect patient privacy and disclose confidential information only with consent of the patient or when required by an overriding duty such as the duty to protect others or to obey the law."[18] Because the law regarding disclosures varies between jurisdictions, emergency physicians should know the law in their jurisdictions and be aware of the underlying ethical tensions in patient confidentiality.[19]

What to Do When Patients Make Threats Against Specific Persons

The requirement for patient confidentiality is not an absolute one. There are established exceptions to this requirement ethically and legally, such as the reporting of certain communicable diseases and the suspected abuse of children or the elderly.[20] Health Insurance Portability and Accountability Act regulations identify 12 national priority purposes that allow disclosure of patient health information as well.[21] An

Table 2	
AIMED strategy proposed by Clark and colleagues[15] for AMA discharges	
Assess	First, assess the severity of the patient's illness and the probable risk of harm that will occur as a result of leaving AMA. Following this determination, assess the patient's decision-making capacity and, if it is impaired, how it might be reversed
Investigate	When investigating the patient's reason for leaving, pay particular attention to potentially modifiable factors influencing this decision, such as level of pain/comfort, presence of withdrawal, and responsibility for the care of others (family or pets). This investigation is also an opportunity to assess the patient's perception of the communication about the condition and treatment plan as well as to try to identify others who the clinician might be able to ally with to address the patient's concerns to help prevent an AMA discharge
Mitigate	If, after the above discussion, patients are still planning to leave AMA, potential further harms should be mitigated by offering treatment alternatives that may be acceptable to the patient, providing prescriptions, aftercare instructions, and a follow-up plan. Choosing to leave AMA should not be seen as the refusal of all medical care and an attempt should be made to identify the maximal level of care the patient is willing to receive/comply with
Explain	Providers should attempt to provide patients with a thorough explanation of the recommended original treatment plan, alternatives, specific potential harms resulting from refusal to follow the recommended plan, and risks and benefits of each. An explicit statement that the patient is welcome to return at any time is also recommended
Document	A best-practice approach to documentation should include a concise description of the patient's condition, proposed and alternative treatments offered, an assessment that the patient was determined to have decision-making capacity, why they refused the proposed treatment, and what care was provided to mitigate the impact of the AMA discharge (negotiation efforts, prescriptions, follow-up plan, and discharge instructions). In addition, it is important to document that the patient received a medical screening examination; the findings of that examination; and, if the patient was unable to be located for a discharge conversation, the efforts to locate them

additional challenging case occurs in emergency psychiatry when a patient makes a threat against an identifiable person. The seminal case of this type occurred in California in 1969 with the murder of Tatiana Tarasoff by Prosenjit Poddar, who had disclosed his intention to kill her to his psychiatrist in advance of the murder. The resulting Supreme Court of California Case established a duty to protect third parties against threatened bodily harm by a patient.[22] Following Tarasoff, significant heterogeneity has developed in states laws through a combination of statutes and court cases, with some states mandating a duty to warn, others permitting a confidentiality breach but not requiring it, and some offering no guidance. In addition, states vary in whether or not these regulations are limited to identifiable victims or any foreseeable victim.[23]

Maintaining the Confidentiality of Psychiatric Patients

Maintaining privacy and confidentially can be challenging in the ED because of the open architecture and high volume of patients.[24] In addition, unauthorized persons are more likely to overhear protected health information in curtained rather than close-walled care spaces.[25] In addition, many psychiatric patients in the ED may require staff to directly observe them to reduce the risk of self-harm or to allow for appropriate staff safety. This requirement can preclude the normal best practice of keeping doors and partitions closed to prevent unauthorized observation.[26] Nonetheless, safety concerns should be balanced against a strong inclination to protect patient privacy and confidentiality because psychiatric conditions can be stigmatizing and evaluation of them often involves the discussion of highly personal information.

A further concern in maintaining the confidentiality of psychiatric patients is the clinical value of obtaining collateral information to formulate an understanding of the patient's condition and to assess dangerousness and safety. Patients should be asked for their permission to talk to family or others but they might refuse. In this case, American Psychiatric Association guidelines support "listening to information provided by family members and other important people in the patient's life, as long as confidential information is not provided to the informant."[27] All staff caring for psychiatric patients should be aware of the need to maintain confidentiality and strive to do so in their practices.

INVOLUNTARY TREATMENT

Involuntary treatment, which is treatment despite a patient's refusal, is fraught with ethical and legal challenges.[28] Involuntary treatment and coercion are negatively associated with patient satisfaction and are commonly experienced by patients who have been admitted to a psychiatric facility.[29] Broad categories of involuntary treatment of relevance to the emergency medicine provider are (1) treatment of emergency medical conditions in patients incapacitated by an acute psychiatric condition; (2) involuntary admission to a mental health facility; (3) testing or medical therapy required to provide medical clearance for psychiatric hospitalization; (4) therapies to control acute behavioral or psychiatric crisis, including medications, seclusion, and restraint. The management of the first category is addressed in the same manner as other instances of incapacity. Involuntary treatment of psychiatric illness that is long term or outside the context of an acute emergency, including long-term medication and electroconvulsive therapy, has its own significant literature basis and jurisdiction specific legal considerations that are outside of the scope of this article.[30] The remaining 3 categories are addressed later.

Involuntary Admission

To admit a patient involuntarily is to deprive that patient of the right to autonomy in the service of beneficence. During involuntary admission, patients are deprived of their autonomy and liberty rights by those in a position of authority; their doctors with the assistance of the state. This deprivation is done with the justification that it is in the patient's best interest and benefit to do so (ie, medical paternalism), or justified by the need to protect society from the individual (ie, social paternalism).[31] Although paternalism has become a pejorative, involuntary admission is an ethically defensible action when used judiciously.[32]

Understanding historical abuses of power through involuntary confinement helps contextualize the current ethical issues in involuntary admission. These abuses included the confinement of the non–mentally ill (eg, Packard v Packard) and the extended confinement of the nondangerous mentally ill (eg, O'Connor v Donaldson); cases that were eventually resolved through litigation. The twentieth century saw a shift in public sentiment and US law regarding civil commitment. Vague statutes with liberal involuntary commitment standards were tightened in the 1970s to protect the civil liberty interests of the mentally ill (eg, Lessard v Schmidt) and the parens patriae model of civil commitment shifted to a police power model, with a standard in most states that required both mental illness and dangerousness as a prerequisite for involuntary admission. Under this system an initial petition is filed by a physician or police officer, providing the clinical basis for an involuntary hold. There is an accompanying legal process in place to protect the liberty interests of the patient in balance with treatment as well as societal and individual protection requirements.[33] Ultimately, involuntary hospitalization is a judicial determination. However, the emergency room assessment is often the first step in that process.

In the modern context, a power differential still remains between doctor and patient because of the physician's expertise and authority, which has the potential for abuse.[34] For example, there is ethical support for the involuntary hospitalization of homicidal patients; however, this authority can blur into the realm of the criminal justice system if these homicidal intentions are not thought to be caused by mental illness. If the goal is to protect others from a threatening person, then anyone with homicidal intent should be detained, regardless of their mental health. However, this is not the purpose of an involuntary hospitalization. Instead, the purpose is to mitigate dangerousness by treating the dangerousness that flows from mental illness, and thereby restore the individual to capacity.[35] Restated, the goal of admission is to protect patients from harm that they would not be exposed to were they capable of autonomous decision making, not dangerous, or not impaired by their psychiatric illness.

Consideration should also be given to whether the proposed benefits of hospitalization clearly outweigh the risks associated with the deprivation of liberty. Patients with dementia, intellectual disability, or severe personality disorders are examples of those who may not be appropriate for commitment, although they may still benefit from admission. These conditions may be subject to such minimal change with acute hospitalization that the benefits of involuntary hospitalization are outweighed by the harm from the deprivation of their rights.[35] For example, in patients with personality disorders, such as borderline personality disorder, there are risks associated with the hospitalization itself, such as fostering behavioral regression or dependence on the hospital for safety, that are not outweighed by the benefits of a brief hospitalization, which are not likely to significantly alter the long-term course of the disorder. However, the hospital would be able to help provide a safe environment for patients who are at imminent risk of harm to themselves or others and could shift the balance toward hospitalization.[36]

What to Do When a Patient Refuses Standard Medical Clearance Testing

The specific role of emergency physicians in the medical evaluation and stabilization of psychiatric patients, commonly referred to as medical clearance, is reviewed separately in this issue.[37] The American College of Emergency Physicians guideline on psychiatric care provides the level B recommendation that "Routine laboratory testing of all patients is of very low yield and need not be performed as part of the ED assessment."[38] An ethical question arises when an emergency physician is asked to perform such testing by a potential accepting psychiatric facility and the patient refuses. The fact that a patient has an acute psychiatric condition requiring involuntary admission does not automatically remove that patient's ability to refuse individual medical and psychiatric tests or treatments. Potential harms to the patient either through delay in receiving psychiatric care or in the physical, emotional, and financial harm of overriding the refusal exist if emergency physicians honor or do not honor this refusal. Determining the nuances of what testing is medically necessary, what the patient has the capacity to refuse, and whether the patient can be transferred without this requested testing is best done by direct communication between the treating emergency physician and the accepting psychiatrist.

Because challenges of this type are likely to recur, this specific concern is an ideal opportunity to institute preventive ethics. Preventive ethics is a term encompassing the strategies of negotiation and respectful persuasion, informed consent as an ongoing process, the use of ethics committees, and the development of institutional policies.[39] An example of a preventive ethics approach addressing this challenge is the formulation of a statewide consensus statement on medical clearance involving a broad partnership of organizations, which occurred in the state of New Jersey. Their statement includes the recommendation that "Patient refusal to consent to a recommended test or procedure shall not result in a delay nor be a reason not to accept a transfer, if a good faith effort is made to obtain consent. This issue should be resolved with physician-to-physician communication."[40] This statement exemplifies the process of preventive ethics and its utility in these types of clinical scenarios rather than to provide a specific recommendation.

Ethical Issues in Forced Medication, Restraint, and Seclusion

The need to address acute behavioral outbursts or safety situations is a key component of the care of emergency psychiatric patients. When possible, collaborative interventions supporting patients' autonomy should be attempted.[41] Behavioral and voluntary medication options may be most supportive of autonomy because they allow patients to have a decision-making role in their treatment. When a patient is overly agitated and collaborative efforts are not possible, treatment of the patient's agitation through forced medication may be considered with the goal of restoration of autonomy, reduced risk of harm, and treatment of the underlying condition. There is also a role for the legitimate self-interests of the care staff in the management of acutely agitated patients because the number of assaults occurring in hospitals has been increasing for several years and continues to be an endemic problem, especially in the ED.[42,43]

When determining intervention, the least invasive means should be tried first. Clinicians can begin with verbal redirection, offering of voluntary medications, intensifying to a show of force, or negotiating reduction in agitation through offerings such as food, beverage, or other assistance. If these are ineffective, emergency medication, physical restraints, or seclusion may be required.[41] In the short term, safety issues are paramount, which may lead to escalating the response sooner rather than later. However, collaboration and less authoritative measures are most favorable for long-term outcomes.[44,45] Previously, treatments for agitation focused on sedation or stupor as the end point of medications for agitation. However, research has shown that sleep is not essential for improvement in agitation or decreasing psychotic symptoms. Thus, the use of medications such as antipsychotics has increased as the end point has shifted toward treatment of the psychosis leading to reduction in agitation.[46] Some of the medications used continue to have a side effect of sedation, and this effect may be beneficial in reducing harm, but it should continue to be viewed as a side effect, not a goal.

Under the Code of Federal Regulations Title 42 Section for Public Health, it is specifically stated that restraints or seclusion may only be imposed to ensure the immediate physical safety of the patient, a staff member, or others and must be discontinued at the earliest possible time.[47] Restraints should be used when all other less restrictive measures to mitigate dangerousness have failed. Restraints are effective in maintaining safety, but are also more difficult to place in the category of treatment because they do not work to improve the patient's underlying condition, and may exacerbate it.[48]

Because restraints and seclusion are more difficult to justify ethically and are less focused on improving the patient's condition compared with ensuring the safety of the emergency room, they should be used for the shortest necessary time and monitored closely throughout.

A question may arise regarding the covert or surreptitious administration of medication to manage a psychiatric emergency. Surreptitious medication administration is different than other types of forced medication because it is through deception that the medication is administered. Lewin and colleagues[49] (2005) described a case report of a bipolar patient administered medication covertly in orange juice to reduce manic symptoms in the ED. The literature is sparse regarding the prevalence of the practice and what is published primarily relates to the nursing home or the institutional setting.[50] The literature is further limited by the secrecy surrounding covert medication because of concern of professional repercussions with the acknowledgment of deceitful prescribing.[51] Some investigators have advocated for further consideration of covert medication in specific circumstances.[52] However, the consideration that surreptitious medication, such as slipping something into a drink, is a less restrictive or superior alternative to physically forcing medication on a patient or risking harm to a patient with a contraindication to restraint must be weighed against the potential disadvantages of surreptitious medication, including denying the patient the opportunity to gain insight, reinforcing the lack of insight into the illness, and violating the trust in the patient-doctor relationship, all of which may deter future help-seeking and treatment acceptance.[31] Because legal and ethical guidelines exist for forced medication, commitment processes, and alternatives to informed consent including assent, covert medication has little established legal or ethical support.

Overall, the key principle in involuntary treatment is to use the least ethically invasive or restricting means available to best support patients' autonomy and interests with the goal of treating the patient's underlying condition and providing a safe environment for the patient and staff.

SUMMARY

The care of patients with a psychiatric emergency is fraught with ethical challenges. Applying ethical reasoning to the clinical challenges of capacity and consent, confidentiality, and involuntary treatment may help to improve care. Emergency providers should be able to assess decision-making capacity using the 4 criteria of communication, understanding, appreciation, and reasoning. When patients are found to be incapacitated, attempts should be made to restore capacity; mitigate harms; and to use surrogates, emergency consent, psychiatric advance directives, and judicial authorization to proceed with care in a situationally appropriate manner. Maintaining patient confidentiality is a strong imperative for emergency physicians and should be protected unless compelling additional concerns take precedence, such as the requirement to follow the law. The goal of involuntary treatment, when used, should be to protect patients from harm that they would not be exposed to were they capable of autonomous decision making, not dangerous, or not impaired by their psychiatric illness using the least restrictive means possible.

REFERENCES

1. Beauchamp TL, Childress JF. Principles of biomedical ethics. 6th edition. New York: Oxford University Press; 2008.

2. Leo RJ. Competency and the capacity to make treatment decisions: a primer for primary care physicians. Prim Care Companion J Clin Psychiatry 1999;1(5): 131–41.

3. Candia PC, Barba AC. Mental capacity and consent to treatment in psychiatric patients: the state of the research. Curr Opin Psychiatry 2011;24:442–6.

4. Raymont V, Bingley W, Buchanan A, et al. Prevalence of mental incapacity in medical inpatients and associated risk factors: cross-sectional study. Lancet 2004;364:1421–7.

5. Buchanan A. Mental capacity, legal competence and consent to treatment. J R Soc Med 2004;97:415–20.

6. Appelbaum PS, Grisso T. Assessing patients' capacities to consent to treatment. N Engl J Med 1988;319:1635–8.

7. Appelbaum PS. Assessment of patients' competence to consent to treatment. N Engl J Med 2007;357:1834–40.

8. Grisso T, Appelbaum PS, Hill-Fotouhi C. The MacCAT-T: a clinical tool to assess patients' capacities to make treatment decisions. Psychiatr Serv 1997;48:1415–9.

9. Chow GV, Czarny MJ, Carrese JA. CURVES: a mnemonic for determining medical decision-making capacity and providing emergency treatment in the acute setting. Chest 2010;137:421–7.

10. Menninger KA. 3rd edition. Advance directives for medical and psychiatric care; in American Jurisprudence Proof of Facts, vol. 102. New York: Thomson Reuters, Lawyers Cooperative Publishing; 2014.

11. Brook M, Hilty DM, Liu W, et al. Discharge against medical advice from inpatient psychiatric treatment: a literature review. Psychiatr Serv 2006;57:1192–8.

12. Kraut A, Fransoo R, Oladson K, et al. A population-based analysis of leaving the hospital against medical advice: incidence and associated variables. BMC Health Serv Res 2013;13:415.

13. Conway KP, Compton W, Stinson FS, et al. Lifetime comorbidity of DSM-IV mood and anxiety disorders and specific drug use disorders: results from the National Epidemiologic Survey on Alcohol and Related Conditions. J Clin Psychiatry 2006; 67:247–57.

14. Hartz SM, Pato CN, Medeiros H, et al. Comorbidity of severe psychotic disorders with measures of substance use. JAMA Psychiatry 2014;71:248–54.

15. Clark MA, Abbott JT, Adyanthaya T. Ethics seminars: a best-practice approach to navigating the against-medical-advice discharge. Acad Emerg Med 2014;21: 1050–7.

16. Kottow MH. Medical confidentiality: an intransient and absolute obligation. J Med Ethics 1986;12:117–22.

17. Veatch R. Case studies in medical ethics. Cambridge (MA): Harvard University Press; 1977. p. 117.

18. American College of Emergency Physicians. Patient Confidentiality. Policy statement reaffirmed October 2008. Available at: http://www.acep.org/Clinical—Practice-Management/Patient-Confidentiality/. Accessed August 30, 2015.

19. McConnell T. Confidentiality and the law. J Med Ethics 1994;20:47–9.

20. Coker R. Tuberculosis, noncompliance and detention for the public health. J Med Ethics 2000;26:157–9.

21. US Department of Health and Human Services, Office for Civil Rights. Standards for privacy of individually identifiable health information; security standards for the protection of electronic protected health information; general administrative requirements including civil monetary penalties: procedures for investigations, imposition of penalties, and hearings. Regulation text. 45 CFR Parts 160 and

164. December 28, 2000 as amended: May 31, 2002, August 14, 2002, February 20, 2003, and April 17, 2003.

22. Tarasoff v Regents of the University of California 551 P 2d 334 9Cal 197.

23. Johnson R, Persad G, Sisti D. The Tarasoff Rule: the implications of interstate variation and gaps in professional training. J Am Acad Psychiatry Law 2014;42: 469–77.

24. Mlinek EJ, Pierce J. Confidentiality and privacy breaches in a university hospital emergency department. Acad Emerg Med 1997;4:1142–6.

25. Barlas D, Sama AE, Ward MF, et al. Comparison of the auditory and visual privacy of emergency department treatment areas with curtains versus those with solid wall. Ann Emerg Med 2001;38:135–9.

26. Moskop JC, Marco CA, Larkin GL, et al. From Hippocrates to HIPPA: privacy and confidentiality in emergency medicine—Part II: challenges in the emergency department. Ann Emerg Med 2005;45:60–7.

27. American Psychiatric Association. Practice guideline for the psychiatric evaluation of adults. 2nd edition. 2006. Available at: http://psychiatryonline.org/pb/assets/raw/sitewide/practice_guidelines/guidelines/psychevaladults.pdf. Accessed March 1, 2015.

28. Wettstein RM. The right to refuse psychiatric treatment. Psychiatr Clin North Am 1999;22:173–82, viii.

29. Strauss JL, Zervakis JB, Stechuchak KM, et al. Adverse impact of coercive treatments on psychiatric inpatients' satisfaction with care. Community Ment Health J 2013;49:457–65.

30. Harris V. Electroconvulsive therapy: administrative codes, legislation, and professional recommendations. J Am Acad Psychiatry Law 2006;34(3):406 11.

31. Kjellin L. Medical and social paternalism: regulation of and attitudes towards compulsory psychiatric care. Acta Psychiatr Scand 1993;88(6):415–9.

32. Derse AR. Law and ethics in emergency medicine. Emerg Med Clin North Am 1999;17(2):307–25.

33. Rosner R, editor. The principles and practice of forensic psychiatry. 2nd edition. Boca Raton (FL): CRC Press. p. 107–12.

34. Geppert CMA. Doctor-patient relationship. Encyclopedia of aging and public health. Springer 2008. p. 288.

35. McLachlan AJ. Criteria for involuntary hospitalisation. Aust N Z J Psychiatry 1999; 33(5):729–33.

36. Miller LJ. Inpatient management of borderline personality disorder. J Personal Disord 1989;3(2):122–34.

37. Tucci V, Siever K, Matorin A, et al. Down the Rabbit Hole: Emergency Department "Medical Clearance" of patients with Psychiatric or Behavioral Emergencies. Emerg Med Clin N Am 2015, in press.

38. Lukens TW, Wolf SI, Edlow JA, et al. Clinical policy: critical issues in the diagnosis and management of the adult psychiatric patient in the emergency department. Ann Emerg Med 2006;46:77–99.

39. Chervenak FA, McCullogh LB. Clinical guides to preventing ethical conflicts between pregnant women and their physicians. Am J Obstet Gynecol 1990;162: 303–7.

40. New Jersey Department of Human Services, Division of Mental Health and Addiction Services. Consensus statement: medical clearance protocols for acute psychiatric patients referred for inpatient admission. 2011. Available at: http://www.nj.gov/humanservices/dmhs/home/Consensus%20Statement%20REVISED%20FINAL%20Apr%2015.pdf. Accessed April 20, 2015.

41. Allen MH, Currier GW, Hughes DH, et al. Treatment of behavioral emergencies: a summary of the expert consensus guidelines. J Psychiatr Pract 2003;9:16–38.

42. Flannery RB, Hanson MA, Penk WE, et al. Hospital downsizing and patients' assaults on staff. Psychiatr Q 1997;68:67–76.

43. Gillespie GL, Gates DM, Berry P. Stressful incidents of physical violence against emergency nurses. Online J Issues Nurs 2013;18(1).

44. Allen MH, Carpenter D, Sheets JL, et al. What do consumers say they want and need during a psychiatric emergency? J Psychiatr Pract 2003;9:39–58.

45. Allen MH, Currier GW, Carpenter D, et al. The expert consensus guideline series: treatment of behavioral emergencies 2005. J Psychiatr Pract 2005;11:5–25.

46. Battaglia J. Pharmacological management of acute agitation. Drugs 2005;65: 1207–22.

47. 42 CFR 482.13 – Condition of participation: patient's rights.

48. Sailas E, Wahlbeck K. Restraint and seclusion in psychiatric inpatient wards. Curr Opin Psychiatry 2005;18:555–9.

49. Lewin MR, Montauk L, Shalit M, et al. An unusual case of subterfuge in the emergency department: covert administration of antipsychotic and anxiolytic medications to control an agitated patient. Ann Emerg Med 2006;47:75–8.

50. Haw C, Stubbs J. Covert administration of medication to older adults: a review of the literature and published studies. J Psychiatr Ment Health Nurs 2010;17: 761–8.

51. Whitty P, Devitt P. Surreptitious prescribing in psychiatric practice. Psychiatr Serv 2000;56:481–3.

52. Hung EK, McNiel DE, Binder RL. Covert medication in psychiatric emergencies: is it ever ethically permissible? J Am Acad Psychiatry Law 2012;40:239–45.

Health Policy Considerations in Treating Mental and Behavioral Health Emergencies in the United States

CrossMark

Thiago C. Halmer, MD, MBA[a],*, Rakel C. Beall, MD[b],
Asim A. Shah, MD[b], Cedric Dark, MD, MPH[a]

KEYWORDS

- Mental health access • ED crowding • Mental health parity • Boarding
- Mental health reform • Substance abuse • Homelessness • Incarceration

KEY POINTS

- The US mental health system, based largely on outpatient services, has failed to meet the growing need for acute psychiatric care in the United States.
- Limited mental health access, especially for acute behavioral emergencies, has led to increased visits in emergency departments (EDs) nationwide.
- The boarding of psychiatric patients in overburdened EDs with inadequately trained staff creates a suboptimal acute care setting that negatively impacts patient care.
- Deficiencies in acute/chronic mental health care have contributed to growing rates of substance abuse, homelessness, and incarceration among the mentally ill in the United States.

HISTORY OF MENTAL HEALTH SERVICES IN THE UNITED STATES

The mental health system in the United States has dramatically evolved in the past 2 centuries. Economic factors, advances in medicine, and changes in government policies have all contributed to a paradigm shift in psychiatric care. During the nineteenth century, the focus in the US mental health policy was to treat those patients who had the most severe and chronic mental health problems. This focus led to the construction of the asylum, a state institution offering shelter and care for those with mental health impairments. Asylums benefited communities, families, and patients alike by

Disclosure statement: The authors have nothing to disclose.
[a] Emergency Medicine, Baylor College of Medicine, 1504 Taub Loop I, Houston, TX 77030, USA;
[b] Psychiatry & Behavioral Sciences, Baylor College of Medicine, Menninger Department of Psychiatry, One Baylor Plaza - BCM350, Houston, TX 77030, USA
* Corresponding author.
E-mail address: thiago.halmer@bcm.edu

Emerg Med Clin N Am 33 (2015) 875–891
http://dx.doi.org/10.1016/j.emc.2015.07.013
0733-8627/15/$ – see front matter © 2015 Elsevier Inc. All rights reserved.

emed.theclinics.com

offering comprehensive therapies and humane custodial care for the chronically ill. By the midnineteenth century, the asylum became widely regarded as a symbol of an "enlightened and progressive nation that no longer ignored or mistreated its insane citizens."[1] By the 1950s, however, positive perceptions of the state mental hospital began to erode as financial neglect, due largely to the Great Depression and World War II, deteriorated the quality of care at these facilities. This deterioration along with several other major developments, including a shift toward psychoanalytic and pharmacologic therapies, an emphasis on preventative approaches, and greater federal government support for community programs, propelled the evolution of the US mental health delivery system virtually overnight. These advances unlocked the doors of state asylums allowing patients to transition into communities for outpatient treatment and management of their psychiatric conditions.

Ultimately, deinstitutionalization of the US mental health system resulted in a decentralized, heterogeneous, community-based array of outpatient services. A mass exodus of psychiatrists from mental hospitals ensued during the late 1950s; by the following decade 80% of the 10,000 members of the American Psychiatric Association were employed outside of mental hospitals.[1] This revolution toward outpatient psychiatry gained momentum with the passage of the National Mental Health Act in 1946 (PL 79-487), which provided federal funding to states to support expanding outpatient care facilities. Beginning in the 1960s, deinstitutionalization resulted in a decrease of beds in state and county psychiatric hospitals. This trend has continued as the number of beds nationwide dropped from approximately 400,000 in 1970 to 50,000 in 2006, with 80% of states reporting a shortage of acute care psychiatric beds.[2,3] Since then, the number of psychiatric hospitals and acute care psychiatric units has maintained a steady decline (**Fig. 1**).

This systemic shift toward prevention and maintenance in outpatient clinics left few options beyond EDs for patients experiencing acute psychiatric exacerbations. Whether due to the long-term effects of deinstitutionalization, inadequate community resources, the large numbers of uninsured patients, or other causes, it is inarguable that the number of patients in psychiatric crises presenting to EDs is on the rise.[4] Between 1992 and 2001, there were 53 million mental-health-related ED contacts in the United States, an increase from 4.9% to 6.3% of all ED visits and an upswing from 17.1 to 23.6 visits per 1000 of the US population during this period.[5] By 2007, psychiatric visits accounted for 12.5% of the 95 million visits to the ED, almost doubling from the proportion (6.3%) in 2001.[4,6]

EMERGENCY MENTAL HEALTH DELIVERY IN THE UNITED STATES TODAY

There are 3 common models of emergency psychiatry delivery in the United States currently differing by where patients are placed.[4] Although each of these models carry their own advantages and disadvantages, the general treatment goals of emergency psychiatry are the same: first exclude medical causes for symptoms, rapidly stabilize the acute crisis, and develop an appropriate disposition and aftercare plan.

Emergency Department Boarding with Psychiatric Consultation

In this traditional model, the patient is evaluated and treated in the ED by both an emergency medicine (EM) physician and a psychiatry consultant. First, the EM physician performs an appropriate medical screening evaluation looking for any organic causes explaining the psychiatric symptoms. Once organic causes are ruled out and/or stabilized, the patient is evaluated by the psychiatry consultant. One major advantage of this model is that it possesses the lowest cost and is the easiest to

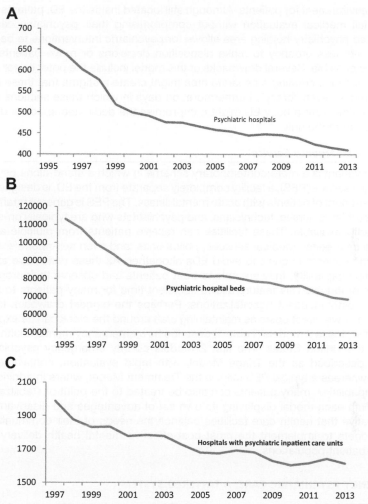

Fig. 1. (*A*) Total number of freestanding psychiatric hospitals in the United States, 1995–2013. (*B*) Total number of beds in US psychiatric hospitals, 1995–2013 (*C*) Total number of US hospitals with inpatient psychiatric units, 1997–2013. (*Adapted from* American Hospital Association. AHA Annual Survey of Hospitals, 1995–2013. AHA Hospital Statistics, 2015 [and earlier] edition.)

implement within most currently existing hospital infrastructures. Potential disadvantages include a delay in diagnosis and interventions depending on when consultants arrive to treat the patient, holding patients in a chaotic ED environment that is not conducive to psychiatric stabilization, and the lack of specialized staff providing psych-specific nursing care for the patient.

Designated Psychiatric Area Within the Emergency Department

Another model that is used in many hospitals involves a separate area within the ED that is dedicated specifically to patients with mental illness. This section is operated by specially trained and dedicated staff focused on creating a more nurturing and calming environment for patients. Although still located inside the ED, patients can still receive full medical evaluation without compromising their psychiatric care. This designated psychiatry holding area allows for psychiatric interventions to be started quickly, with less urgency to make disposition decisions or move patients out as quickly as possible. Several drawbacks of this model include the potential for marginalization because creating a separate area might create a stigma that these patients are different or even "crazy". Furthermore, on days in which these sections are less used, overflow from a busy ED might compromise the dedicated space and/or float staff away from the unit.

Psychiatric Emergency Service

The third variant is a more contemporary scheme in which a stand-alone psychiatric emergency service (PES), a facility completely separate from the ED, is designed solely for the treatment of patients with acute mental illness. The PES is generally staffed 24 h/d with psychiatric nurses, technicians, and psychiatrists who are typically on-site or at least readily available. These facilities can receive patients from multiple avenues, including emergency medical services, police units, and even self-referrals, allowing psychiatric patients in crisis to avoid EDs altogether. As these units have extended observation capability, they are able to treat patients and observe their progress for 24-hours or longer. This feature allows sufficient time for many patients to stabilize avoiding costly inpatient hospitalizations. Perhaps the biggest drawback from this model is its own direct costs as maintaining staff around the clock can be expensive.

Together, these 3 models (**Table 1**) describe how emergency mental health is practiced in the United States. The first 2 models portray emergency psychiatry in a method described as the Triage Model, with rapid evaluation, containment, and referral, whereas a typical PES follows the Treatment Model, where in addition to triaging capabilities, many patients can also be treated to the point of stabilization on-site.[4,7] With each model displaying its own set of advantages and disadvantages, it is imperative that health care facilities balance the needs of their communities with their budgets to implement the most cost-effective mental health delivery system for their patient populations.

EMERGENCY PSYCHIATRIC CARE: A TATTERED SYSTEM

According to a *USA Today* special report in 2014, more than half a million Americans with serious mental illness are falling through the cracks of a "mental health system in tatters."[8] With a dearth of mental health access points nationwide, these patients have nowhere to go during acute psychiatric decompensation and often fall hard in EDs, jails, or city streets. Consequently, EDs have become the principal acute care site in the US mental health system, wherein psychiatrists and EM physicians are working together to keep a sinking ship afloat.

There has been a recent shift in US health care toward quality assurance, cost-effectiveness, and improved health outcomes. This shift coupled with rising public awareness and concern after mental-health-related mass violence has led to growing calls for mental health reform. With emergency rooms now becoming the epicenters for psychiatric and behavioral emergencies, increased scrutiny of psychiatric public policy has led to closer analysis of the major issues surrounding this sector of US health care. Some of the most pressing issues outside the emergency room include inadequate to no mental health coverage for patients, dwindling investment in the field of psychiatry, and insufficient psychiatric access both in terms of care providers and psychiatric hospital beds. These dilemmas have contributed to various problems

Table 1
Common models of emergent psychiatric care in the United States

	Care Model	Description	Advantages	Disadvantages
Triage Models	Psychiatric care in ED	Patients with mental illness housed, evaluated, and treated by psychiatry consultant in general ED	• Possesses the lowest cost and is the easiest to implement within most currently existing hospital infrastructures	• Delay in definitive diagnosis and intervention • Chaotic setting not conducive to psychiatric stabilization • Lack specialized nursing care • Potential for marginalization in separating psychiatric patients
	Psychiatric section in ED	Separate section within ED with specialized staff dedicated to evaluation and treatment of mental health patient	• Specialized staff creating a more nurturing and calming care area • Allows psychiatric interventions to start immediately	
Treatment Model	Psychiatric emergency service	Stand-alone psychiatric unit with specialized staff used solely to evaluate, treat, and stabilize patients in mental health crisis	• Immediately treat for 24 h or longer to stabilize avoiding costly inpatient hospitalizations	• High costs of maintaining specialized staff around the clock

Adapted from Zeller SL. Treatment of psychiatric patients in emergency settings. Prim Psychiatry 2010;17(6):35–41.

within the ED including overcrowding, increased boarding of psychiatric patients, lack of specialized staff treating the acutely ill psychiatric patient, and diminished workplace safety for ED providers and staff. Together, these deficiencies in mental health delivery have led to even greater societal problems including increased mental-health-related violence, elevated incarceration rates, increased drug abuse and dependency, and worsening homelessness. By recognizing these deficiencies and confronting them head-on in a collaborative manner, providers and policymakers will be able to create innovative, multidisciplinary solutions to the delivery of acute mental health emergencies.

TREATING MENTAL AND BEHAVIORAL HEALTH EMERGENCIES: MENTAL HEALTH SYSTEM CONSIDERATIONS
Inadequate Mental Health Coverage

Perhaps one of the core problems of the US health care system is inadequate patient funding. Despite steady reductions in the number of uninsured Americans since implementation of the Affordable Care Act (ACA) of 2010 (P.L. 111–148, P.L. 111–152), there are still 38 million Americans lacking any type of health insurance.[9] It has been shown that adults with mental illness lack coverage at significantly higher rates than those without mental illness.[10] According to a recent survey of patients with psychiatric conditions, 61% of those not receiving mental health care listed cost as a barrier (**Fig. 2**).[11] Consequently, these patients may seek care in EDs.

For vulnerable populations, Medicaid, a federal-state social health care program, covers comprehensive care for mental illness and substance abuse. Medicaid eligibility is based on federally established minimums for states to cover certain population groups such as low-income adults, seniors, pregnant women, children, and those with disabilities. At present, states have the option to implement their own eligibility criteria as long as they are within the federally mandated minimums. In 2013, more than 62 million Americans were covered by Medicaid.[12] Medicaid is the largest mental health payer accounting for approximately 28% of all mental health spending in the United States ($32 billion in 2005) (**Fig. 3**).[13] It subsidizes care for millions of low-income Americans with conditions such as schizophrenia, bipolar disorder, substance abuse, and other severe psychiatric disorders.[14]

Originally, the ACA mandated that all US citizens and legal residents with income up to 133% of the poverty line, including adults without dependent children, would qualify for coverage in any state that participated in the Medicaid program. However, in National *Federation of Independent Business v Sebelius*, the US Supreme Court ruled that states will have the option to adopt this expansion or continue with their pre-ACA eligibility standards.[15] With only 26 states now participating, 10.6 million people living in states opting out of this expansion are not eligible for Medicaid expansion, leaving approximately 3.7 million mental health patients without health insurance or access to mental health services.[16] Previous estimates that 20% to 40% of emergency psychiatry visits are unnecessary[17] implies that the refusal of some states to adopt the ACA Medicaid expansion might contribute to overuse of the ED for acute psychiatric care when outpatient settings might be more appropriate.

Pharmacologic treatments remain first-line, evidence-based treatments for most major mental illnesses and represent approximately one-fifth of Medicaid mental health spending.[18,19] Many states have implemented cost containment strategies aimed at reducing these prescription drug costs. These strategies include prior authorization requirements, preferred drug lists, step therapy policies (ie, covering a nonpreferred medication only after documented failure of payer-preferred medications), limits

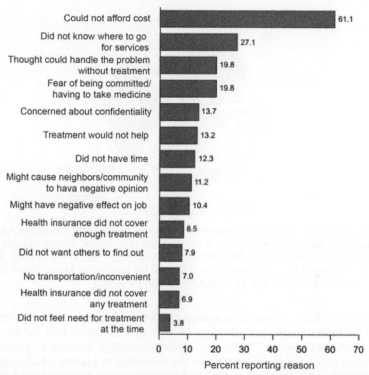

Fig. 2. Reasons for not receiving mental health services in the past year among adults aged 18 years or older with past year any mental illness and a perceived unmet need for mental health care who did not receive mental health services. (*From* Substance Abuse and Mental Health Services Administration. Results from the 2013 National Survey on Drug Use and Health: Mental Health Findings, NSDUH Series H-49, HHS Publication No. (SMA) 14-4887. Rockville (MD): Substance Abuse and Mental Health Services Administration; 2014.)

on the number of prescriptions that can be filled in a month, and requirements to use generics.[14] Some states are attempting to increase patient copayments in an effort to reduce health care spending.[20] While these policies might help reduce pharmaceutical expenditures, they can create obstacles for patients trying to initiate and maintain their recommended medication regimens. Studies have shown that these policies may result in medication discontinuations, gaps, and switches, leading to unfavorable patient outcomes and increased nondrug health care use (eg, ED visits, hospitalizations), potentially offsetting any pharmaceutical savings.[14]

Limitations in mental health coverage apply to private insurance plans as well. In fact, historically even those insured by private third-party payers and/or employers have been impacted by inadequate coverage. For instance, there has been a lack of parity between how insurance companies cover psychiatric versus medical care. Historically, coverage for mental health care has had its own cost-sharing (usually higher) structure, more restrictive limits on inpatient stay and outpatient visits, annual and lifetime caps, and different prior authorization requirements than coverage for other medical care.[21] Cumulatively, this has made mental health coverage far less generous than coverage for medical care. Legislations such as the Mental Health Parity Act of 1996 (PL 104-204) and the Mental Health Parity and Addiction Equity Act

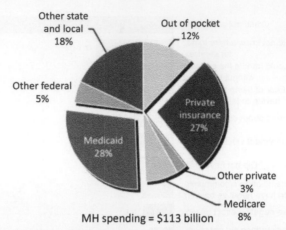

Fig. 3. Spending on mental health treatment by payer, 2005. (*From* Substance Abuse and Mental Health Services Administration. National Expenditures for Mental Health Services and Substance Abuse Treatment, 1986–2005. DHHS Publication No. (SMA) 10-4612. Rockville (MD): Center for Mental Health Services and Center for Substance Abuse Treatment, Substance Abuse and Mental Health Services Administration; 2010.)

(MHPAEA) of 2008 (PL 110-343) have aimed to fix this problem by prohibiting differences in treatment limits, cost sharing, as well as in-network and out-of-network coverage between mental health and general medical insurance. Notably, the MHPAEA has extended these policies to the treatment of substance use disorders. It is estimated that 62.5 million people with behavioral and substance abuse disorders will benefit from parity protections.[22]

Diminished Investment in Psychiatric Care

A case can be made that the United States is not allocating enough resources toward psychiatric care. Despite spending a total of $113 billion on mental health,[23] the US health care system is not addressing the growing unmet treatment needs of its psychiatric populations. In fact, 89% of the 24 million people aged 12 years and older with a substance use or dependence disorder received no specialty treatment of their condition in 2006.[24] Of the 33 million adults aged 18 years and older needing mental health treatment, 31% received inadequate care or no care at all.[25] At the same time, the United States is experiencing its largest increase in adolescent suicide rates in more than a decade, an indication that those most in need are not being treated.[26]

Overall, mental health spending has grown more slowly than general health spending, despite the increased rate of use of care services since the 1970s.[27] However, state and federal policymakers often view mental health resources as expendable, especially when constrained by budget limitations; this is especially true during recessions when policymakers tend to attribute their budget woes to out-of-control mental health spending.[27] For example, during the most recent recession from 2008 to 2011, states cut 1.8 billion from their mental health budgets (**Fig. 4**).[28]

One significant impact of these cuts is that much of the treatment of the mentally ill shifts toward other access points in the health care system. For example, after a series of budget cuts from 2008 to 2011, Rhode Island saw a 65% increase in the number of children with mental illness seeking care in EDs.[28] As noted by Frank and Glied,[27] 2006, "the future growth in mental health spending could be constrained by the cost containment strategies of public policymakers." In order to change this trend,

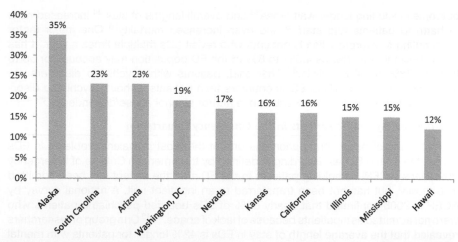

Fig. 4. Largest mental health state budget cuts as a percentage of overall state general fund for mental health services, 2009–2011. (*Data from* National Alliance on Mental Health (NAMI). State mental health cuts: a national crisis. 2011. Available at: https://www2.nami. org/ContentManagement/ContentDisplay.cfm?ContentFileID=125018. Accessed March 23, 2015.)

constituencies will need to convey a greater sense of urgency in this matter to help propel mental health as a top priority in political and health policy agendas.

Diminished Access to Psychiatric Care

In the past 60 years, most psychiatric care in the United States has transitioned from long-term public hospitals to privatized acute care facilities. In an effort to reduce costs, states have drastically downsized state hospitals, shifting the psychiatric cost burden to the federal government (ie, Medicaid) and private insurers. There has been a steady decline and now shortage of psychiatric beds in the United States. For example, in 1990 there were more than 50,000 beds in general hospital psychiatric units across the country and 45,000 beds in private psychiatric hospitals.[3] By 2002, there were only 25,000 private psychiatric hospital beds and 40,000 general hospital beds.[29] During this same period, psychiatric visits to the emergency room increased from 1.4 million to nearly 2.5 million in 2003.[30]

Managed care tactics have reduced reimbursement rates making it difficult even for outpatient facilities to operate. This has led to shortfalls in funding for community-based services, causing many outpatient practices to close their doors. For example, a report by the Minnesota Psychiatric Society noted that one organization in the state closed 6 of its 9 outpatient clinics because of inadequate payments.[31] As the number of inpatient psychiatric beds has decreased, the dwindling resources for outpatient services have not kept up with the demand. Essentially, this barrier to access contributes to more cases of decompensated psychiatric disease, increasing the number of preventable ED visits.

TREATING MENTAL AND BEHAVIORAL HEALTH EMERGENCIES: EMERGENCY DEPARTMENT POLICY CONSIDERATIONS

EDs across the United States are becoming increasingly crowded, with many frequently operating beyond capacity. In 2010, the number of annual ED visits nationwide was estimated to be 129.8 million and rising.[32] ED crowding can lead to negative outcomes including longer wait times[33] and overall lengths of stay,[34] increased risks of harm to patients and staff,[35] and even increased mortality[36] One major factor contributing to overcrowding is patients who revisit EDs multiple times a year. It has been shown that as few as 4.5% to 8% of the ED population may account for up to 21% to 28% of all ED visits.[37] That said, patients with psychiatric disorders are more likely to have multiple ED encounters than patients without psychiatric disorders,[38] particularly if they have substance and/or alcohol abuse/dependency.[39–41]

Boarding of Psychiatric Patients in the Emergency Department

The boarding of psychiatric patients is one of the most prevalent problems in EDs across the United States. Boarding is defined by the American College of Emergency Physicians (ACEP) as holding patients in the ED after the patient has been admitted to a facility, but has not been transferred to an inpatient unit. A national survey by ACEP in 2008 confirmed that nearly 80% of EDs boarded psychiatric patients who were not admitted as inpatients because of lack of space.[42,43] One group of researchers revealed that the average length of stay in EDs is 42% longer for patients with mental health problems, averaging more than 11 hours nationally.[44] In another study, 1 in 12 patients with psychiatric complaints had an ED length of stay of greater than 24 hours.[43]

Perhaps one of the most overt reasons for the extended ED boarding of psychiatric patients is the dwindling availability of psychiatric hospital beds in the United States. Patients can be held in the ED for hours to days before a bed becomes available for them in a psychiatric unit. One retrospective case-control study found 4 characteristics strongly associated with length of stay in excess of 24 hours including suicidal ideation, homicidal ideation, need for inpatient admission, and a lack of insurance (**Box 1**).[45]

Other reasons include the length of time it takes for some patients, especially those who are acutely agitated or intoxicated, to return to full cognitive functioning and achieve clinical stability. Furthermore, those who are acutely agitated and impeding their own care may require pharmacologic sedation, further delaying psychiatric evaluation until these patients return to their cognitive baseline. During this time, patients are kept in their ED beds indefinitely, many times delaying any definitive psychiatric interventions until they can be medically cleared.

There have been several proposals to help decrease boarding in EDs nationwide; however, more research is needed to validate the impact that they will have. First and foremost, access to outpatient and inpatient psychiatric care needs to improve. Increased state and federal funding should be used to improve access to the mental health system with an emphasis on creating additional avenues for services. One interesting proposal is to establish benchmarks in the ED care of psychiatric patients, such as measuring the number of visits lasting greater than 24 hours.[43] This statistic could be used as a quality metric directly tied to hospital reimbursement rates, incentivizing

---

Box 1
Characteristics associated with length of stays greater than 24 hours

- Suicidal ideation
- Homicidal ideation
- Need for inpatient admission
- Lack of insurance

Data from Park JM, Park LT, Siefert CJ, et al. Factors associated with extended length of stay for patients presenting to an urban psychiatric service: a case-control study. J Behav Health Serv Res 2009;36:300–8.

hospitals to address this problem. Furthermore, concurrent medical and psychiatric evaluation instead of a stepwise evaluation protocol can easily reduce delays in treating psychiatric patients in the ED.[46] Together, these systemic improvements could substantially decrease ED boarding and improve the level of care hospitals provide to their communities.

Lack of Specialized Staff for Psychiatric Patients in the Emergency Department

To exacerbate the issue of boarding, ED staff may lack adequate understanding of mental illness or even harbor negative sentiments toward psychiatric patients. ED staff often report a sense of fear and anger provoked by the aggressive or bizarre behavior many of these patients present with.[47] In addition, the revolving door nature of many presentations along with poor follow-up care and medication nonadherence results in a sense of hopelessness and a why bother attitude in staff.[48] One study found that the greater the negative affect of staff toward the patient who is mentally ill, the less the propensity to help.[48]

Many ED health professionals do not receive adequate training in caring for patients with mental illness; they often lack the deescalation skills and safety techniques that can assure a safe environment for themselves and the patient. Without these skills, ED staff often prematurely jump to the use of restraints, seclusion, and/or sedatives, which can further deteriorate a patient's condition or delay definitive evaluation. In consequence, this can increase the length of stay of patients and in some instances lead to unnecessary hospital admissions.

There is a dire need to better train ED staff to provide a higher level of care to patients in acute mental health crisis. It has been postulated that patients who receive higher-quality initial care are more likely to go home than stay in the emergency room as boarders.[49] For example, hospitals that participated in the Institute for Behavioral Healthcare Improvement's 2008 learning collaborative, a national initiative to improve behavioral health, found that they were able to reduce the length of stay of psychiatric patients in the ED and the use of seclusion and restraints with low-cost interventions including improved training for clinical and security staff.[49] By training staff in deescalation techniques, they were able to significantly reduce boarding times and improve patient experiences.[49] Since the number of psychiatric emergencies presenting to EDs will likely not subside anytime soon, it would be prudent to consider instituting national psychiatric training standards for all ED care providers.

TREATING MENTAL HEALTH EMERGENCIES: POLICY CONSIDERATIONS BEYOND THE HOSPITAL
Drug Abuse and Dependence in Mental Illness

Mental illness and substance abuse are highly comorbid conditions. Estimates based on past studies reveal that alcohol and drug dependence are twice as common among individuals with anxiety disorders, affective disorders, and psychotic disorders.[50] Statistics from the 2013 National Survey on Drug Use and Health indicate that close to 7.7 million adults in the United States have both mental and substance use disorders (**Fig. 5**).[51]

In another study, patients with severe mental illness were about 4 times more likely to be heavy alcohol users (4 or more drinks per day), 3.5 times more likely to use marijuana regularly (21 times per year), and 4.6 times more likely to use other drugs at least 10 times in their lives.[50] One reason for this is the tendency of these patients to self-medicate with alcohol and/or drugs to treat their psychiatric symptoms. Patients with mental health disorders are seeking treatment of substance abuse and/or intoxication

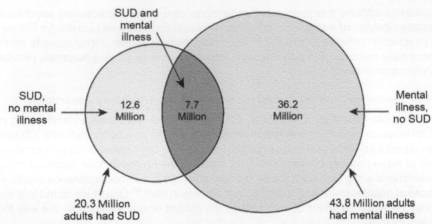

SUD and
mental
illness

SUD,
no mental
illness

12.6
Million

7.7
Million

36.2
Million

Mental
illness,
no SUD

20.3 Million
adults had SUD

43.8 Million adults
had mental illness

Fig. 5. Past year substance abuse and mental illness among adults aged 18 years or older. SUD, substance use disorder. (*From* Substance Abuse and Mental Health Services Administration. Results from the 2013 National Survey on Drug Use and Health: Mental Health Findings, NSDUH Series H-49, HHS Publication No. (SMA) 14-4887. Rockville (MD): Substance Abuse and Mental Health Services Administration; 2014.)

in EDs at an increasing rate. One study in Maryland reviewing data from 2008 to 2012 showed that the prevalence of co-occurring mental illness among substance-abuse-related encounters increased from 53% to 57% for ED encounters.[52] This trend creates serious problems for an already vulnerable population and will continue as long as these patients continue to lack proper access to long-term psychiatric care.

There have been some promising developments in the treatment of substance abuse with the advent of the ACA. This law establishes the treatment of addiction and behavioral disorders as a mandatory coverage in all health care plans. The law has also increased the integration of substance abuse treatment into general medical settings, including the ED. These changes will help EDs go beyond just screening and stabilizing patients and offer initial treatments and direct referrals so that patients can continue their care once discharged. Although these initiatives have helped address the previous inadequacies in the treatment of substance abuse, it will likely increase the number of ED visits in the short term. More needs to be done to increase outpatient access for patients for both mental health and substance abuse disorders.

Mental Illness and Homelessness

According to the Substance Abuse and Mental Health Services Administration, 20% to 25% of the homeless population in the United States has some form of severe mental illness. Serious mental illness disrupts patients' ability to care for themselves, including finding employment, managing daily responsibilities, and forming stable and supportive relationships, resulting in them becoming homeless. A study of people with serious mental illnesses seen by California's public mental health system found that 15% were homeless at least once in a 1-year period.[53]

The National Alliance to End Homelessness estimates that there were approximately 250,000 homeless persons with serious mental illnesses in the United States, following steady increases since the 1970s. This growing trend is not only evident in major cities but also in small cities and towns across the nation. For example, in Roanoke, Virginia, this population increased 363% between 1987 and 2007, with 70% of the homeless population receiving mental health treatment at some point in their past. As the mentally ill continue to lack the adequate care they need, more and more of these patients will be forced to live on the streets.

It is important to consider all aspects of patient living when treating mental health disorders. In a world with endless resources, the care of these patients would be comprehensive with provisions to also provide housing and employment services to help psychiatrically compensated patients reintegrate back into society. One important first step is to improve community access to long-term psychiatric care. In addition, increased capacity in psychiatric hospitals can help fully stabilize and treat acute exacerbations of mental illness before these patients turn to substance abuse to cope with their disorders.

Incarceration of the Mentally Ill

In a 2006 special report, the Bureau of Justice Statistics estimated that 705,600 mentally ill adults were incarcerated in State prisons, 78,800 in federal prisons, and 479,900 in local jails.[54] Research suggests that "people with mental illnesses are overrepresented in probation and parole populations at estimated rates ranging from two to four times the general population."[55] This fact has caused significant strain on US law enforcement agencies and correctional facilities for several reasons. First, individuals with mental illness are jailed on an average 2 to 3 times longer than individuals without a mental illness arrested for a similar crime.[56] Next, jails incur significant costs associated with the oversight of prisoners with mental illness for medication and other health care services.[56] Last, these inmates have very little chance of rehabilitation while incarcerated without proper psychiatric care; this increases the likelihood that they will remain a danger to society or become repeat offenders. Moreover, a stay in jail may even exacerbate the person's illness and at the very least tarnish his or her public record making it more difficult to regain employment and reintegrate back into the society.[56]

Medication nonadherence is a major reason why psychiatric patients decompensate and begin acting erratically and/or commit crimes. In one study, it was shown that monthly medication possession and receipt of outpatient services reduced the likelihood of any arrests.[57] This study further concluded that there was "an additional protective effect against arrest for individuals in possession of their prescribed pharmacological medications for 90 days after hospital discharge."[57] Thus, increasing community access to outpatient psychiatric services after incarceration should be the cornerstone of any mental health reform.

There is also a clear link between mental illness, homelessness, drug abuse, and incarceration. Many homeless psychiatric patients are arrested for nonviolent crimes including trespassing, petty theft, or possession of illegal substances. About 74% of state prisoners and 76% of local jail inmates who had a mental health problem met criteria for substance dependence or abuse.[58] Public policies addressing homelessness and improved care modalities for substance abuse disorders will go a long way toward diminishing incarceration rates of those with mental illness.

SUMMARY

The US mental health system has evolved drastically with care shifting from institutionalization of patients to a more community-based outpatient treatment. Today, limited funding and access, especially for the uninsured and for those in acute psychiatric crisis, have plagued this outpatient care system; this in turn has led to an increase in psychiatric care visits in EDs across the United States. With decreasing inpatient psychiatric bed availability, the boarding of psychiatric patients in EDs often delays definitive treatments and ties up hospital resources even negatively impacting the care of others. Consequently, the suboptimal mental health care that these patients receive has led to even broader societal issues including increases in substance abuse and intoxication, homelessness, and incarceration rates. Although there are several proposals on how to improve the mental health care system, there has been very little action. The time has come for health providers and policymakers to come together and implement an action plan to improve the care for millions of mental health patients in the United States.

REFERENCES

1. Grob GN. Mental health policy in America: myths and realities. Health Aff (Millwood) 1992;11(3):7–22.
2. Tuttle GA. Report of the Council on Medical Service, American Medical Association: access to psychiatric beds and impact on emergency medicine. Chicago: AMA; 2008.
3. Sharfstein SS, Dickerson FB. Hospital psychiatry for the twenty-first century. Health Aff 2009;28(3):685–8.
4. Zeller SL. Treatment of psychiatric patients in emergency settings. Prim Psychiatry 2010;17(6):35–41.
5. Larkin GL, Claassen CA, Emond JA, et al. Trends in U.S. emergency department visits for mental health conditions, 1992 to 2001. Psychiatr Serv 2005;56(6):671–7.
6. Chang G, Weiss AP, Orav J, et al. Bottlenecks in the emergency department: the psychiatric clinicians' perspective. Gen Hosp Psychiatry 2012;34:403–9.
7. Gerson S, Bassuk E. Psychiatric emergencies: an overview. Am J Psychiatry 1980;137(1):1–11.
8. Szabo L. Cost of not caring: nowhere to go. USA Today 2015. Available at: http://www.usatoday.com/story/news/nation/2014/05/12/mental-health-system-crisis/7746535. Accessed February 22, 2015.
9. Martinez ME, Cohen RA. Health insurance coverage: early release of estimates from the National Health Interview Survey, January–June 2014. Hyattsville (MD): National Center for Health Statistics; 2014. Available at: http://www.cdc.gov/nchs/nhis/releases.htm. Accessed February 3, 2015.
10. Garfield L. Mental health financing in the United States, a primer. Menlo Park (CA): The Kaiser Commission on Medicaid and the Uninsured; 2011. Available at: https://kaiserfamilyfoundation.files.wordpress.com/2013/01/8182.pdf. Accessed January 28, 2015.
11. Substance Abuse and Mental Health Services Administration. Results from the 2009 National Survey on Drug Use and Health: Volume I. Summary of National Findings (Office of Applied Studies, NSDUH Series H-38A, HHS Publication No. SMA 10-4856 Findings). Rockville (MD): 2010.
12. The Henry J. Kaiser Family Foundation. Medicaid: a primer. Menlo Park (CA): The Kaiser Commion on Medicaid and the Uninsured; 2013. Available at: https://kaiserfamilyfoundation.files.wordpress.com/2010/06/7334-05.pdf. Accessed February 21, 2015.
13. Substance Abuse and Mental Health Services Administration. National expenditures for mental health services and substance abuse treatment, 1986–2005. DHHS publication no. (SMA) 10-4612. Rockville (MD): Center for Mental Health Services and Center for Substance Abuse Treatment, Substance Abuse and Mental Health Services Administration; 2010.
14. West JC, Rae DS, Huskamp HA, et al. Medicaid medication access problems and increased psychiatric hospital and emergency care. Gen Hosp Psychiatry 2010;32:615–22.

15. National Federation of Independent Business v Sebelius, 567 U. S. Case No: 11-393 (2012).

16. Ollove M. Nearly 4 million seriously mentally ill still without insurance. Kaiser health news nearly 4 million seriously mentally ill still without insurance. Washington, DC: Kaiser Family Foundation: Kaiser Health News; 2014. Available at: http:// kaiserhealthnews.org/news/stateline-mental-health. Accessed March 15, 2015.

17. Zeman L, Arfken CL. Decreasing unnecessary care in a psychiatric emergency service. Psychiatr Serv 2006;57(1):137–8.

18. American Psychiatric Association. Practice guidelines for the treatment of psychiatric disorders compendium. Arlington (VA): American Psychiatric Association; 2006.

19. Bergman D, Hoadley J, Kaye N, et al. Using clinical evidence to manage pharmacy benefits: experiences of six states. Issue Brief (Commonw Fund) 2006; 899:1–14.

20. Smith V, Gifford K, Ellis E, et al. Headed for a crunch: an update on Medicaid spending, coverage and policy heading into an economic downturn: results from a 50-state Medicaid budget survey for state fiscal years 2008 and 2009. Menlo Park (CA): Kaiser Commission on the Uninsured; 2008. Available at: http://www.kff.org/medicaid/7815. Accessed February 21, 2015.

21. Goodell S. Health policy brief: mental health parity. Bethesda (MD): Health Affairs; 2014. Available at: http://www.healthaffairs.org/healthpolicybriefs/brief.php?brief_id=112. Accessed December 2, 2014.

22. Beronio K, Po R, Skopec L, et al. Affordable Care Act will expand mental health and substance use disorder benefits and parity protections for 62 million Americans. Washington, DC: HHS, Office of the Assistant Secretary for Planning and Evaluation; 2013. Available at: http://aspe.hhs.gov/health/reports/2013/mental/rb_mental.cfm. Accessed February 20, 2015.

23. Mark TL, Levit KR, Vandivort-Warren R, et al. Changes in US spending on mental health and substance abuse treatment, 1986– 2005, and implications for policy. Health Aff 2011;30(2):284–92.

24. Substance Abuse and Mental Health Services Administration. "Need and receipt of specialty treatment," Sec. 7.3 in 2006. Rockville (MD): National Survey on Drug Use and Health; 2008. Available at: https://www.asipp.org/documents/2006NSDUH.pdf. Accessed December 15, 2014.

25. Substance Abuse and Mental Health Services Administration. "Adults aged eighteen or older," Sec. 8.1 in 2006. Rockville (MD): National Survey on Drug Use and Health; 2008. Available at: https://www.asipp.org/documents/2006NSDUH.pdf. Accessed December 15, 2014.

26. Centers for Disease Control and Prevention. CDC Report Shows Largest One-Year Increase in Youth Suicide Rate in Fifteen Years. CDC Newsroom; 2007. Available at: http://www.cdc.gov/media/pressrel/2007/r070906.htm. Accessed February 2, 2015.

27. Frank RG, Glied S. Changes in mental health financing since 1971: implications for policymakers and patients. Health Aff (Millwood) 2006;25(3):601.

28. National Alliance on Mental Health (NAMI). State mental health cuts: a national crisis. 2011. Available at: https://www2.nami.org/ContentManagement/ContentDisplay.cfm?ContentFileID=125018. Accessed March 23, 2015.

29. Foley DJ, Manderscheid RW, Atay JE, et al. Highlights of Organized Mental Health Services in 2002 and Major National and State Trends in Mental Health, United States, 2004. In: Manderscheid RW, Berry JT, editors. Rockville (MD): Substance Abuse and Mental Health Services Administration; 2006. p. 200–36.

30. Salinsky E, Loftis C. Shrinking Inpatient psychiatric capacity: cause for celebration or concern? NHPF Issue Brief 2007;823:1–21.
31. Minnesota Psychiatric Society. Task force report: the shortage of psychiatrists and of inpatient psychiatry bed capacity. St Paul (MN): MPS; 2002.
32. Centers for Disease Control and Prevention. Atlanta (GA): National Hospital Ambulatory Medical Care Survey. 2010.
33. Hing E, Bhuiya F. Wait time for treatment in hospital emergency departments: 2009. NCHS data brief, No. 102. Hyattsville (MD): National Center for Health Statistics; 2012.
34. McCarthy M, Zeger S, Ding R, et al. Crowding delays treatment and lengthens emergency department length of stay, even among high-acuity patients. Ann Emerg Med 2009;54:492–503.
35. Moskop JC, Sklar DP, Geiderman JM, et al. Emergency department crowding, part 2—barriers to reform and strategies to overcome them. Ann Emerg Med 2009;53(5):612–7.
36. Sun B, Hsia R, Weiss R, et al. Effect of emergency department crowding on outcomes of admitted patients. Ann Emerg Med 2013;61:605–11.
37. LaCalle E, Rabin E. Frequent users of emergency departments: the myths, the data, and the policy implications. Ann Emerg Med 2010;56:42–8.
38. Baillargeon J, Thomas C, Williams B, et al. Medical emergency department utilization patterns among uninsured patients with psychiatric disorders. Psychiatr Serv 2008;59:808–11.
39. Chaput Y, Lebel M. Demographic and clinical profi les of patients who make multiple visits to psychiatric emergency services. Psychiatr Serv 2007;58:335–41.
40. Curran G, Sullivan G, Williams K, et al. Emergency department use of person with comorbid psychiatric and substance abuse disorders. Ann Emerg Med 2003;41:659–67.
41. Minassian A, Vilke G, Wilson M. Frequent emergency department visits are more prevalent in psychiatric, alcohol abuse, and dual diagnosis conditions than in chronic viral illnesses such as hepatitis and human immunodeficiency virus. J Emerg Med 2013;45:520–5.
42. ACEP Psychiatric and substance abuse survey 2008. Washington, DC: American College of Emergency Physicians; 2008.
43. Chang G, Weiss A, Kosowsky JM, et al. Characteristics of adult psychiatric patients with stays of 24 hours or more in the emergency department. Psychiatr Serv 2012;63(3):283–6.
44. McCullumsmith C, Clark B, Blair C, et al. Rapid follow-up for patients after psychiatric crisis. Community Ment Health J 2015;51:139–44.
45. Park JM, Park LT, Siefert CJ, et al. Factors associated with extended length of stay for patients presenting to an urban psychiatric service: a case-control study. J Behav Health Serv Res 2009;36:300–8.
46. Zun LS. Pitfalls in the care of the psychiatric patient in the emergency department. J Emerg Med 2012;43(5):829–35.
47. Clarke D, Usick R, Sanderson A, et al. Emergency department staff attitudes towards mental health consumers: a literature review and thematic content analysis. Int J Ment Health Nurs 2014;23:273–84.
48. Mackay N, Barrowclough C. Accident and emergency staff's perceptions of deliberate self-harm: attributions, emotions and willingness to help. Br J Clin Psychol 2005;44:255–67.
49. Alakeson V, Pande N, Ludwig M. A plan to reduce emergency room 'boarding' of psychiatric patients. Health Aff 2010;29(9):1637–42.

50. Hartz SM, Pato CN, Medeiros H, et al. Comorbidity of severe psychotic disorders with measures of substance use. JAMA Psychiatry 2014;71(3):248–54.
51. Substance Abuse and Mental Health Services Administration. Results from the 2013 national survey on drug use and health: mental health findings, NSDUH series H-49, HHS publication No. (SMA) 14-4887. Rockville (MD): Substance Abuse and Mental Health Services Administration; 2014.
52. Huang TJ, Yang J, Moyo P, et al. Co-occurring mental illness in emergency department and hospital inpatient encounters related to substance abuse in Maryland. Addict Sci Clin Pract 2015;10(Suppl 1):A22.
53. Folsom DP, Hawthorne W, Lindamer L, et al. Prevalence and risk factors for homelessness and utilization of mental health services among 10,340 patients with serious mental illness in a large public mental health system. Am J Psychiatry 2005;162:370–6.
54. Sabol WJ, Couture H, Harrison PM. Prisoners in 2006. Bureau of Justice statistics bulletin 2006: Bureau of Justice statistics. Washington, DC: U.S. Department of Justice Office of Justice Programs; 2007. Available at: http://www.bjs.gov/content/pub/pdf/p06.pdf. Accessed March 15, 2015.
55. Prins S, Draper L. Improving outcomes for people with mental illnesses under community corrections supervision: a guide to research-informed policy and practice. New York: Council of State Governments Justice Center; 2009.
56. Petrila J, Redlich A. Mental illness and the courts: some reflections on judges as innovators. Court Review 2008;43:163–76.
57. VanDorn RA, Desmarais SL, Haynes D, et al. Effects of outpatient treatment on risk of arrest of adults with serious mental illness and associated costs. Psychiatr Serv 2013;64:856–62.
58. James DJ, Glaze LE. Mental health problems of prison and jail inmates. Washington, DC: U.S. Dept. of Justice, Office of Justice Programs, Bureau of Justice Statistics; 2006.

Index

Note: Page numbers of article titles are in **boldface** type.

Emerg Med Clin N Am 33 (2015) 893–899
http://dx.doi.org/10.1016/S0733-8627(15)00086-3
0733-8627/15/$ – see front matter © 2015 Elsevier Inc. All rights reserved.

United States Postal Service

Statement of Ownership, Management, and Circulation
(All Periodicals Publications Except Requestor Publications)

1. Publication Title Emergency Medicine Clinics of North America	2. Publication Number 0 0 0 - 7 1 1 4	3. Filing Date 9/18/15
4. Issue Frequency Feb, May, Aug, Nov	5. Number of Issues Published Annually 4	6. Annual Subscription Price $315.00

7. Complete Mailing Address of Known Office of Publication (Not printer) (Street, city, county, state, and ZIP+4®)

Elsevier Inc.
360 Park Avenue South
New York, NY 10010-1710

Contact Person
Stephen R. Bushing

Telephone (Include area code)
215-239-3688

8. Complete Mailing Address of Headquarters or General Business Office of Publisher (Not printer)

Elsevier Inc., 360 Park Avenue South, New York, NY 10010-1710

9. Full Names and Complete Mailing Addresses of Publisher, Editor, and Managing Editor (Do not leave blank)

Publisher (Name and complete mailing address)

Linda Belfus, Elsevier Inc., 1600 John F. Kennedy Blvd., Suite 1800, Philadelphia, PA 19103

Editor (Name and complete mailing address)

Patrick Manley, Elsevier Inc., 1600 John F. Kennedy Blvd., Suite 1800, Philadelphia, PA 19103-2899

Managing Editor (Name and complete mailing address)

Adrianne Brigido, Elsevier Inc., 1600 John F. Kennedy Blvd., Suite 1800, Philadelphia, PA 19103-2899

10. Owner (Do not leave blank. If the publication is owned by a corporation, give the name and address of the corporation immediately followed by the names and addresses of all stockholders owning or holding 1 percent or more of the total amount of stock. If not owned by a corporation, give the names and addresses of the individual owners. If owned by a partnership or other unincorporated firm, give its name and address as well as those of each individual owner. If the publication is published by a nonprofit organization, give its name and address.)

Full Name	Complete Mailing Address
Wholly owned subsidiary of	1600 John F. Kennedy Blvd. Ste. 1800
Reed/Elsevier, US holdings	Philadelphia, PA 19103-2899

11. Known Bondholders, Mortgagees, and Other Security Holders Owning or Holding 1 Percent or More of Total Amount of Bonds, Mortgages, or Other Securities. If none, check box ▸ ☐ None

Full Name	Complete Mailing Address
N/A	

12. Tax Status (For completion by nonprofit organizations authorized to mail at nonprofit rates) (Check one)
The purpose, function, and nonprofit status of this organization and the exempt status for federal income tax purposes:
☐ Has Not Changed During Preceding 12 Months
☐ Has Changed During Preceding 12 Months (Publisher must submit explanation of change with this statement)

13. Publication Title Emergency Medicine Clinics of North America	14. Issue Date for Circulation Data Below August 2015

15.	Extent and Nature of Circulation	Average No. Copies Each Issue During Preceding 12 Months	No. Copies of Single Issue Published Nearest to Filing Date
a.	Total Number of Copies (Net press run)	738	606
b. Legitimate Paid and/Or Requested Distribution (By Mail and Outside the Mail)	(1) Mailed Outside County Paid/Requested Mail Subscriptions stated on PS Form 3541. (Include paid distribution above nominal rate, advertiser's proof copies and exchange copies)	372	299
	(2) Mailed In-County Paid/Requested Mail Subscriptions stated on PS Form 3541. (Include paid distribution above nominal rate, advertiser's proof copies and exchange copies)		
	(3) Paid Distribution Outside the Mails Including Sales Through Dealers And Carriers, Street Vendors, Counter Sales, and Other Paid Distribution Outside USPS®	128	147
	(4) Paid Distribution by Other Classes of Mail Through the USPS (e.g. First-Class Mail®)		
c.	Total Paid and/or Requested Circulation (Sum of 15b (1), (2), (3), and (4))	500	446
d. Free or Nominal Rate Distribution (By Mail and Outside the Mail)	(1) Free or Nominal Rate Outside-County Copies included on PS Form 3541	72	73
	(2) Free or Nominal Rate In-County Copies included on PS Form 3541		
	(3) Free or Nominal Rate Copies mailed at Other classes Through the USPS (e.g. First-Class Mail®)		
	(4) Free or Nominal Rate Distribution Outside the Mail (Carriers or Other means)		
e.	Total Nonrequested Distribution (Sum of 15d (1), (2), (3) and (4))	72	73
f.	Total Distribution (Sum of 15c and 15e)	572	519
g.	Copies not Distributed (See instructions to publishers #4 (page #3))	166	87
h.	Total (Sum of 15f and g)	738	606
i.	Percent Paid and/or Requested Circulation (15c divided by 15f times 100)	87.41%	85.93%

* If you are claiming electronic copies go to line 16 on page 3. If you are not claiming Electronic copies, skip to line 17 on page 3

16. Electronic Copy Circulation	Average No. Copies Each Issue During Preceding 12 Months	No. Copies of Single Issue Published Nearest to Filing Date
a. Paid Electronic Copies		
b. Total paid Print Copies (Line 15c) + Paid Electronic copies (Line 16a)		
c. Total Print Distribution (Line 15f) + Paid Electronic Copies (Line 16a)		
d. Percent Paid (Both Print & Electronic copies) (16b divided by 16c X 100)		

☐ I certify that 50% of all my distributed copies (electronic and print) are paid above a nominal price

17. Publication of Statement of Ownership
If the publication is a general publication, publication of this statement is required. Will be printed in the **November 2015** issue of this publication.

18. Signature and Title of Editor, Publisher, Business Manager, or Owner

Stephen R. Bushing

Date
September 18, 2015

Stephen R. Bushing – Inventory Distribution Coordinator

I certify that all information furnished on this form is true and complete. I understand that anyone who furnishes false or misleading information on this form or who omits material or information requested on the form may be subject to criminal sanctions (including fines and imprisonment) and/or civil sanctions (including civil penalties).

PS Form 3526, July 2014 (Page 1 of 3 (Instructions Page 3)) PSN: 7530-01-000-9931 PRIVACY NOTICE: See our Privacy policy in www.usps.com

PS Form 3526, July 2014 (Page 3 of 3)

Moving?

Make sure your subscription moves with you!

To notify us of your new address, find your **Clinics Account Number** (located on your mailing label above your name), and contact customer service at:

Email: **journalscustomerservice-usa@elsevier.com**

800-654-2452 (subscribers in the U.S. & Canada)
314-447-8871 (subscribers outside of the U.S. & Canada)

Fax number: 314-447-8029

Elsevier Health Sciences Division
Subscription Customer Service
3251 Riverport Lane
Maryland Heights, MO 63043

*To ensure uninterrupted delivery of your subscription, please notify us at least 4 weeks in advance of move.

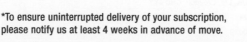

Printed and bound by CPI Group (UK) Ltd, Croydon, CR0 4YY

03/10/2024

01040465-0019